Surgery

Editor

COURTNEY FANKHANEL

PHYSICIAN ASSISTANT CLINICS

www.physicianassistant.theclinics.com

Consulting Editor
JAMES A. VAN RHEE

April 2021 • Volume 6 • Number 2

ELSEVIER

1600 John F. Kennedy Boulevard • Suite 1800 • Philadelphia, Pennsylvania, 19103-2899

http://www.theclinics.com

PHYSICIAN ASSISTANT CLINICS Volume 6, Number 2
April 2021 ISSN 2405-7991, ISBN-13: 978-0-323-75777-5

Editor: Katerina Heidhausen
Developmental Editor: Axell Ivan Jade Purificacion

Physician Assistant Clinics (ISSN: 2405–7991) is published quarterly by Elsevier Inc., 360 Park Avenue South, New York, NY 10010-1710. Months of issue are January, April, July, and October. Periodicals postage paid at New York, NY and additional mailing offices. Subscription prices are $150.00 per year (US individuals), $290.00 (US institutions), $100.00 (US students), $150.00 (Canadian individuals), $297.00 (Canadian institutions), $100.00 (Canadian students), $150.00 (international individuals), $297.00 (international institutions), and $100.00 (international students). Foreign air speed delivery is included in all *Clinics* subscription prices. All prices are subject to change without notice. POSTMASTER: Send address changes to *Physician Assistant Clinics*, Elsevier Periodicals Customer Service, 11830 Westline Industrial Drive, St. Louis, MO 63146. Customer Service Health Sciences Division, Subscription Customer Service, 3251 Riverport Lane, Maryland Heights, MO 63043. **Customer Service: 1-800-654-2452 (U.S. and Canada); 314-447-8871 (outside U.S. and Canada). Fax: 314-447-8029. E-mail: journalscustomerservice-usa@elsevier.com (for print support); journalsonlinesupport-usa@elsevier.com (for online support).**

Reprints. For copies of 100 or more, of articles in this publication, please contact the Commercial Reprints Department, Elsevier Inc., 360 Park Avenue South, New York, NY 10010-1710. Tel. 212-633-3874; Fax: 212-633-3820; E-mail: reprints@elsevier.com.

Physician Assistant Clinics is covered in *EMBASE/Excerpta Medica and ESCI*.

PROGRAM OBJECTIVE
The goal of the Physician Assistant Clinics is to keep practicing physician assistants up to date with current clinical practice by providing timely articles reviewing the state of the art in patient care.

TARGET AUDIENCE
Physician Assistants and other healthcare professionals

LEARNING OBJECTIVES
Upon completion of this activity, participants will be able to:
1. Review the role of PAs in the intra-hospital peri-operative environment.
2. Discuss how PAs can contribute to outpatient pre- and post-surgical evaluations and care.
3. Recognize the roles PAs can play in various surgical subspecialties.

ACCREDITATION
The Elsevier Office of Continuing Medical Education (EOCME) is accredited by the Accreditation Council for Continuing Medical Education (ACCME) to provide continuing medical education for physicians.

The EOCME designates this journal-based CME activity for a maximum of 12 *AMA PRA Category 1 Credit*(s)™. Physicians should claim only the credit commensurate with the extent of their participation in the activity.

All other healthcare professionals requesting continuing education credit for this enduring material will be issued a certificate of participation.

DISCLOSURE OF CONFLICTS OF INTEREST
The EOCME assesses conflict of interest with its instructors, faculty, planners, and other individuals who are in a position to control the content of CME activities. All relevant conflicts of interest that are identified are thoroughly vetted by EOCME for fair balance, scientific objectivity, and patient care recommendations. EOCME is committed to providing its learners with CME activities that promote improvements or quality in healthcare and not a specific proprietary business or a commercial interest.

The planning committee, staff, authors and editors listed below have identified no financial relationships or relationships to products or devices they or their spouse/life partner have with commercial interest related to the content of this CME activity:
Rebecca Arko, MMSc, PA-C; Emily Barber, MHS, PA-C; Carey L. Barry, MHS, PA-C, MT(ASCP); Esther Bennitta; Gayle B. Bodner, MMS, PA-C; Brennan Bowker, MHS, PA-C, CPAAPA; Rebecca Orsulak Calabrese, MHS, PA-C, CPAAPA; Regina Chavous-Gibson, MSN, RN; Amanda C. Chi, MD; Kristi A. Collins, MS, PA-C; Andrew P. Dhanasopon, MD; Elizabeth C. Erickson, MS, PA-C; Courtney Fankhanel, PA-C, MMSc; Katerina Heidhausen; Margaret H. Holland, MSHS, PA-C; Bri Kestler, PA-C, MMS; Holly H. Kim, MD; Kayla McLaughlin, PA-C; Melissa M. Poh, MD; Angela Preda, PA-C; Axell Ivan Jade Purificacion; Polina Reyblat, MD; Rita A. Rienzo, MMSc, PA-C; Elizabeth M. Roessler, MMSc, PA-C; Erin L. Sherer, EdD, PA-C, RD; Mary Showstark, MPAS, PA-C; James A. Van Rhee, MS, PA-C; Holly Zurich, PA-C

UNAPPROVED/OFF-LABEL USE DISCLOSURE
The EOCME requires CME faculty to disclose to the participants:
1. When products or procedures being discussed are off-label, unlabelled, experimental, and/or investigational (not US Food and Drug Administration [FDA] approved); and
2. Any limitations on the information presented, such as data that are preliminary or that represent ongoing research, interim analyses, and/or unsupported opinions. Faculty may discuss information about pharmaceutical agents that is outside of FDA-approved labelling. This information is intended solely for CME and is not intended to promote off-label use of these medications. If you have any questions, contact the medical affairs department of the manufacturer for the most recent prescribing information.

TO ENROLL
The CME program is available to all Physician Assistant Clinics subscribers at no additional fee. To subscribe to the Physician Assistant Clinics, call customer service at 1-800-654-2452 or sign up online at www.physicianassistant.theclinics.com.

METHOD OF PARTICIPATION
In order to claim credit, participants must complete the following:
1. Complete enrolment as indicated above

2. Read the activity
3. Complete the CME Test and Evaluation. Participants must achieve a score of 70% on the test. All CME Tests and Evaluations must be completed online

CME INQUIRIES/SPECIAL NEEDS

For all CME inquiries or special needs, please contact elsevierCME@elsevier.com.

Contributors

CONSULTING EDITOR

JAMES A. VAN RHEE, MS, PA-C
Associate Professor, Program Director, Yale School of Medicine, Yale Physician Assistant Online Program, New Haven, Connecticut

EDITOR

COURTNEY FANKHANEL, PA-C, MMSc
Assistant Professor, Yale Physician Associate Program, Physician Assistant, Cardiac Surgery, Yale New Haven Hospital, New Haven, Connecticut

AUTHORS

REBECCA ARKO, MMSc, PA-C
Physician Assistant, Cardiac Surgery, Yale New Haven Hospital, New Haven, Connecticut

EMILY BARBER, MHS, PA-C
Physician Assistant Program, Quinnipiac University, Hamden, Connecticut

CAREY L. BARRY, MHS, PA-C, MT(ASCP)
Program Director and Assistant Clinical Professor, Physician Assistant Program, Bouvé College of Health Sciences, Northeastern University, Boston, Massachusetts

GAYLE B. BODNER, MMS, PA-C
Assistant Professor, Department of Anesthesiology and PA Studies, Wake Forest School of Medicine, Winston-Salem, North Carolina

BRENNAN BOWKER, MHS, PA-C, CPAAPA
Senior Surgical Physician Assistant, Department of Surgery, Emergency and General Surgery, Yale New Haven Hospital, Part-Time Clinical Assistant Professor of Physician Assistant Studies, Quinnipiac University, Department of Physician Assistant Studies, New Haven, Connecticut

REBECCA ORSULAK CALABRESE, MHS, PA-C, CPAAPA
Surgical Float Physician Assistant, Department of Surgery, Yale New Haven Hospital, New Haven, Connecticut

AMANDA C. CHI, MD
Department of Urology, Kaiser Permanente, Los Angeles, California

KRISTI A. COLLINS, MS, PA-C
Assistant Professor, Master of Physician Assistant Studies Program, Franklin Pierce University, West Lebanon, New Hampshire

ANDREW P. DHANASOPON, MD
Assistant Professor, Department of Surgery, Section of Thoracic Surgery, Yale University, New Haven, Connecticut

ELIZABETH C. ERICKSON, MS, PA-C
Physician Assistant with Trauma/General Surgery, MidMichigan Medical Center, Midland, Michigan

COURTNEY FANKHANEL, PA-C, MMSc
Assistant Professor, Yale Physician Associate Program, Physician Assistant, Cardiac Surgery, Yale New Haven Hospital, New Haven, Connecticut

MARGARET H. HOLLAND, MSHS, PA-C
Surgical Physician Assistant, Department of Cardiac Surgery, Boston Children's Hospital, Boston, Massachusetts

BRI KESTLER, PA-C, MMS
Simulation Program, University of South Alabama, Mobile, Alabama

HOLLY H. KIM, MD
Transition Pathways Clinic, Kaiser Permanente, Los Angeles, California

KAYLA MCLAUGHLIN, PA-C
Department of Plastic Surgery, Kaiser Permanente, Los Angeles, California

MELISSA M. POH, MD
Department of Plastic Surgery, Kaiser Permanente, Los Angeles, California

ANGELA PREDA, PA-C
Physician Assistant, Smilow Cancer Hospital, Yale New Haven Hospital, New Haven, Connecticut

POLINA REYBLAT, MD
Department of Urology, Kaiser Permanente, Los Angeles, California

RITA A. RIENZO, MMSc, PA-C
Assistant Professor and Director of Clinical Education, Yale School of Medicine Physician Associate Program, New Haven, Connecticut

ELIZABETH M. ROESSLER, MMSc, PA-C
Assistant Professor and Director of Didactic Education, Yale School of Medicine Physician Associate Program, New Haven, Connecticut

ERIN L. SHERER, EdD, PA-C, RD
Emergency Department Physician Assistant, Columbia University Irving Medical Center, New York, New York

MARY SHOWSTARK, MPAS, PA-C
Assistant Professor Adjunct, Physician Assistant Online Program, Yale School of Medicine, New Haven, Connecticut

HOLLY ZURICH, PA-C
Lead Advanced Practice Provider, Performance Improvement Surgical Services, Yale New Haven Health, New Haven, Connecticut

Contents

Ordering preoperative testing for patients undergoing noncardiac surgery should be considered on a case-by-case basis. For most patients, ordering laboratory studies and other preoperative assessments provides little benefit for risk stratification or improving postoperative outcomes. Preoperative studies should be considered only after a thorough history and physical examination have been undertaken and then only if the results would alter perioperative management.

Postoperative ileus (POI) is a transient impairment of bowel function that commonly occurs after intra-abdominal surgery. Although it is an often-expected outcome after major surgery, it not only causes significant morbidity to the patient but also increases length of stay and hospital costs exponentially. Recently, there has been a greater focus on decreasing POI incidence; this has been achieved through enhanced recovery after surgery pathways. By increasing use of nonopioid pain modalities, feeding patients sooner, and focusing on early ambulation, rates of POI have decreased.

Periprosthetic joint infection is a rare, devastating complication. Common symptoms include persistent wound drainage, joint effusion, fever, acute/chronic joint pain, persistent stiffness, or decreased range of motion. Prompt diagnosis is critical for effective treatment. The preoperative workup includes a serum erythrocyte sedimentation rate and C-reactive protein, serum D-dimer, synovial fluid culture, synovial fluid cell counts with differential, synovial fluid leukocyte esterase, alpha-defensin testing, and synovial fluid erythrocyte sedimentation rate. A new diagnostic algorithm using has been developed to aid diagnosis. Once diagnosed, treatment may include debridement, antibiotics, irrigation and retention of implants; single-stage or 2-stage revision, and targeted antibiotics.

environments working with limited resources. Working in disaster surgery takes teamwork, dedication, and perseverance.

Carey L. Barry

Surgical site infections are among of the most common hospital acquired infections. Surgical site classification, evaluation, diagnosis, and treatment are reviewed. Current guidelines for surgical site infection prevention are summarized.

Rebecca Arko and Courtney Fankhanel

Aortic stenosis (AS) is the most common valvular heart disease in the western world, accounting for 43% of all single, native, left-sided valve disease. The disease is more common in the elderly population and continues to increase in prevalence as the population ages. Consequently, the health care system must prepare for the growing number of patients with AS who necessitate an aortic valve replacement. Clinicians should be aware of the symptoms and physical examination findings patients may experience as a result of AS, as well as the appropriate management and escalation of care.

Bri Kestler

Chronic venous insufficiency is a common vascular disorder and develops from persistent venous hypertension. Leg pain, edema, varicose veins, and skin changes are the most common clinical manifestations of venous disease. Socioeconomic consequences include impaired social engagement, loss of work hours because of disabling symptoms, diminished quality of life, and financial burden to patients and the health care system. Conservative therapy includes lifestyle changes, leg elevation, and the use of compression hose to counter increased venous hydrostatic pressures. Interventional management varies from sclerotherapy for spider, reticular, and varicose veins, to endovenous thermal ablation for closure of incompetent saphenous veins.

Gayle B. Bodner

Respiratory concerns in the perioperative setting are common and costly and impact patient morbidity and mortality. Predictors of pulmonary complications are multifaceted, including components of time, acuity, patient-specific risk factors, and often, most important, characteristics of the surgery. These concerns can arise acutely during the perioperative course in patients with or without chronic comorbidities. Preoperative assessment is ideal for risk stratification, medical optimization, and planning for postoperative monitoring and management.

Video content accompanies this article at http://www. physicianassistant.theclinics.com.

Even as community awareness of gender dysphoria and insurance coverage for transgender medicine increases, education regarding gender-affirming care remains sparse for health care providers. Gender-affirming genitourinary surgery complications span from minor to requiring multiple surgical interventions and may present in the primary care setting. This article provides a review of genitourinary gender-affirming surgeries and associated complications.

PHYSICIAN ASSISTANT CLINICS

SERIES OF RELATED INTEREST

Surgical Clinics
http://www.surgical.theclinics.com/
Medical Clinics
http://www.medical.theclinics.com/

THE CLINICS ARE AVAILABLE ONLINE!
Access your subscription at:
www.theclinics.com

Foreword
COVID

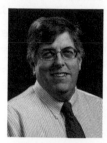

James A. Van Rhee, MS, PA-C
Consulting Editor

By the time this issue is published, I hope we are deep into the distribution of a COVID-19 vaccine. These have been trying times: separated from family and friends, loss of loved ones, and the daily feeling of unease during the pandemic. But it is hoped these new vaccines will change the effect this virus has on our lives. I hope we will feel normal again with the vaccine. In the future, when someone coughs or sneezes, I hope the first thing we think about is not COVID. In the future, when we see someone wearing a surgical mask on the street, I hope our thoughts do not go immediately to COVID. In the future, when we are in a crowded room or at a sporting event, I hope we will stop wondering if someone near me has COVID. Let us hope we can soon get back to the days of enjoying cultural and sporting events, dining out with friends, and spending time with patients without personal protective equipment. Thank you to all the health care providers, who have sacrificed so much to care for all patients, both with and without COVID. I hope, when things get back to some sense of normalcy, we can honor all the providers the way they deserve to be honored.

This issue of *Physician Assistant Clinics*, with guest editor, Courtney Fankhanel, provides an excellent review of several topics in surgery. These will benefit the surgical and nonsurgical physician assistant (PA). For the surgical PA, Zurich and Preda provide a comprehensive review of chest tubes, and with the assistance of Dhanasopan, Zurich and Preda also review chest tube drainage in the age of COVID-19. Sherer provides a discussion of enhanced recovery after surgery, and Showstark reviews disaster surgery. Bodner reviews perioperative respiratory concerns, and McLaughlin, Poh, Chi, Reyblat, and Kim discuss gender-affirming genitourinary surgery.

For the surgical and nonsurgical PA, Rienzo and Roessler discuss preoperative evaluation for noncardiac surgery; Bowker, Orsulak, and Barber review postoperative ileus, and Collins describes periprosthetic joint infections. Barry describes surgical wound infections; Fankhanel discusses aortic stenosis, and Kestler reviews chronic venous insufficiency.

Physician Assist Clin 6 (2021) xiii–xiv
https://doi.org/10.1016/j.cpha.2021.01.002
2405-7991/21/© 2021 Published by Elsevier Inc.

physicianassistant.theclinics.com

I hope you enjoy this issue. Our next issue will cover topics in behavioral health.

James A. Van Rhee, MS, PA-C
Yale School of Medicine
Yale Physician Assistant Online Program
100 Church Street South, Suite A230
New Haven, CT 06519, USA

E-mail address:
james.vanrhee@yale.edu

Website:
http://www.paonline.yale.edu

Preface
Surgery

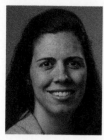

Courtney Fankhanel, PA-C, MMSc
Editor

The mainstay of physician assistant (PA) training continues to be generalist in nature; however, once certified, many go on to choose careers in surgery and various surgical subspecialties. Surgical PAs are trained to provide care in the entire spectrum of the perioperative environment, including preoperative/preadmission care, intraoperative assisting and expertise, postoperative care in a variety of surgical intensive care units, stepdown units, postanesthesia care units, and surgical floors. In addition to the multiple intrahospital roles surgical PAs contribute to, many also provide presurgical and postsurgical outpatient evaluations and care. It is an ever-growing and complex role for the PA profession that offers many the opportunity to practice at the top of their license.

This publication of *Physician Assistant Clinics* is dedicated to a broad range of surgical topics spanning from preoperative evaluation, postoperative complications, enhanced recovery guidelines, to background information and important topics within the subspecialties of orthopedic, thoracic, cardiac, vascular, trauma, and plastic surgery. It is my hope that this issue provides its readers with important information they can use to help enhance their own care of patients in any practice setting.

Courtney Fankhanel, PA-C, MMSc
Yale Physician Associate Program
PO Box 208083
New Haven, CT 06520-8083

E-mail address:
courtney.fankhanel@yale.edu

Physician Assist Clin 6 (2021) xv
https://doi.org/10.1016/j.cpha.2021.01.001
2405-7991/21/© 2021 Published by Elsevier Inc.

physicianassistant.theclinics.com

Preoperative Evaluation for Noncardiac Surgery

Rita A. Rienzo, MMSc, PA-C*, Elizabeth M. Roessler, MMSc, PA-C

KEYWORDS

- Surgery • Physician assistant • Preoperative care • Preoperative laboratory testing
- Testing protocols

KEY POINTS

- Preoperative testing should include a focused history and physical examination, with a thorough review of the patient's medical record and guided by the risk of the proposed procedure.
- Avoid testing in low-risk surgical candidates who are having minimal risk or minimally invasive surgical procedures. It often is unnecessary to repeat recently obtained tests unless there has been some change in overall clinical condition.
- Given the lack of specific testing guidelines, there often is excessive ordering of both diagnostic and laboratory tests, leading to false-positive results and without significant change in clinical outcomes.

INTRODUCTION

An estimated 48.3 million surgical and nonsurgical procedures are performed annually in hospital and ambulatory surgery centers.[1] Prior to undergoing a surgical procedure, many patients are referred to their primary care physician assistant for a preoperative evaluation. According to the American Board of Internal Medicine (ABIM) Choosing Wisely campaign, the goal of the preoperative evaluation is to identify, stratify, and reduce risk for major postoperative complications.[2] The crucial elements of this evaluation include a careful history and physical examination. Preoperative testing for low-risk surgical procedures typically does not reclassify the risk estimate established through the history and physical examination. Additionally, the goal of the preoperative assessment is not solely to give routine medical clearance for surgery but also to provide comprehensive guidance on perioperative evaluation and management, including risk stratification and optimization.[3] The provider should consider 3 guiding questions when evaluating a patient for surgery: What is the patient's risk of complications? Would further risk stratification alter the surgical management of this patient?

Yale University School of Medicine Physician Associate Program, PO Box 208083, New Haven, CT 06520-8083, USA
* Corresponding author.
E-mail address: RITA.RIENZO@YALE.EDU

Physician Assist Clin 6 (2021) 209–213
https://doi.org/10.1016/j.cpha.2020.11.001
2405-7991/21/© 2020 Elsevier Inc. All rights reserved.

and Can the patient's risk be reduced?[4] Despite the recommendations of the ABIM, many patients still undergo routine testing. In addition to the benefits of a thorough history and physical examination, this article reviews the most commonly requested laboratory and diagnostic testing.

THE MEDICAL HISTORY AND PHYSICAL EXAMINATION

The medical history and physical examination in a preoperative evaluation are among the most important tools PAs have and can provide guidance in decisions about diagnostic imaging and laboratory testing. Additionally, these components can help identify individuals who may be a risk for perioperative or postoperative complications.

The Medical History

A complete review of systems is necessary to identify any undiagnosed disease or poorly controlled chronic disease, such as pulmonary or cardiac issues that potentially may contribute to poor surgical outcomes. The social history discloses any current or remote tobacco or substance use disorders. An extensive medication history should be obtained to include over-the-counter or herbal supplements as well as recent use of nonsteroidal anti-inflammatory drugs (NSAIDs), anticoagulants, or aspirin products, which may prolong bleeding time. Medication allergies, especially to antibiotics, or allergies to latex products or to foods associated with latex sensitivities (such as apricots, avocados, bananas, chestnuts, and kiwis) need to be documented. A detailed surgical and anesthetic history should be obtained. Family history may reveal coagulopathy, cardiac disease, or other pathology that requires further investigation. A reaction to anesthesia by the patient or by family members raises concerns about a predisposition to malignant hypothermia. Such a risk requires a consultation by an anesthesiologist and specific equipment in the surgical suite.

The Physical Examination

The physical examination should build on the information gathered during the medical history. Along with documentation of vital signs, all patients should receive a thorough oropharyngeal, cardiovascular, and pulmonary examinations. In addition, any positive findings elicited in the review of systems should be evaluated further, especially recent infections, bleeding dyscrasias, or recent cough or fever.

ROUTINE LABORATORY STUDIES

One of the 5 major goals of the Choosing Wisely initiative was to "to identify tests or procedures commonly used...whose necessity should be questioned and discussed."[2] Numerous reviews of the existing data subsequently were undertaken to determine the utility of routine preoperative laboratory studies in identifying unrecognized risk factors in otherwise healthy patients undergoing low-risk surgery. There was little evidence to suggest that results from routine studies were fundamental to perioperative management or significantly improved outcomes.[5,6] Current practice guidelines recommend that routine preoperative testing for low-risk surgeries be driven by medical necessity based on history and physical examination rather than institutional protocols.[5,7]

Coagulation Studies

Coagulation studies, usually defined as prothrombin time, partial thromboplastin time, and international normalized ratio, should not be performed routinely on patients in the absence of any indication of coagulopathy. As discussed previously, a thorough patient and family history is the most effective means of determining the likelihood of a bleeding disorder[7]; therefore, such testing should be reserved for patients whose history suggests underlying liver disease (or risk factors for such, including alcohol abuse disorder), malnutrition, previous bleeding disorders, easy bruising, or other pathology that potentially could interfere with hemostasis. A history of anticoagulant drug therapy, such as warfarin, or NSAID use also must be elicited, along with a family history of coagulopathy or bleeding, in particular, excessive surgical bleeding. On physical examination, note the presence of bruises or petechiae that may suggest underlying coagulopathy.[4] The rationale behind this guidance is that the prevalence of undetected bleeding disorders is low, and the most common one, von Willebrand disease, is not detectable by routine coagulation studies.[8]

Complete Blood Cell Count

The need for hemoglobin and hematocrit levels preoperatively depends on several factors. Because patients with preoperative values outside the normal range are at a higher risk for adverse outcomes postoperatively, patients at risk of anemia or polycythemia or with a history of liver disease or other hematologic disorders should be screened. Patients at the extremes of age also should be tested,[7,9] as should patients undergoing complex or major surgery.[10]

Additionally, the likelihood of significant blood loss should be discussed with the surgeon. In those cases where blood loss could be significant or the need for transfusion may arise, the availability of preoperative hemoglobin and hematocrit levels helps guide postoperative management.

A white blood cell count should be obtained if ongoing inflammation or occult infection is suspected.

Electrolytes and Creatinine

Although electrolytes and renal function measurements are ordered routinely as part of a preoperative evaluation, no trials have documented changes in postoperative outcomes among patients who had electrolyte screening prior to surgical procedures.[3] Guidance in screening should be determined by findings on patient-specific history and physical examination, in particular those findings related to heart failure, chronic kidney disease, and diabetes. Use of certain medications, such as diuretics, angiotensin-converting enzyme inhibitors, angiotensin II receptor blockers, and NSAIDs, should inform decisions to perform presurgical electrolyte and creatinine testing.

Glucose and Hemoglobin A_{1c}

There is no clear agreement that supports routine preoperative glucose or glycated hemoglobin testing in healthy patients. This lack of guidance is in contrast to the significant body of evidence that demonstrates a clear association between perioperative hyperglycemia and adverse clinical outcomes.[11] Blood glucose testing should be obtained if there is a clinical suspicion of potential disturbances in glucose metabolism or if the patient is at risk for diabetes. Additionally, for patients undergoing surgeries that have an increased risk of infectious complications, such as vascular, orthopedic, or spinal procedures, or complex intra-abdominal surgeries, routine testing for blood glucose might be justified.

Urinalysis

There is no evidence supporting routine urinalysis in asymptomatic patients without clinical suspicion. A case series has shown that abnormalities were seen in up to

34% of patients but these results led to a change in management less than 14% of the time and of those patients fewer than 1% had postoperative complications.[5] Guideline consensus is that routine urinalysis is not recommended in asymptomatic patients except those undergoing surgical implantation of foreign material, such as heart valves or joint replacements, or invasive urogynecological procedures.[6]

ELECTROCARDIOGRAM

A screening electrocardiogram (ECG) often is ordered as part of a preoperative evaluation, yet the routine diagnostic value is unclear. Guidelines state a routine ECG is not useful and does not have an impact on outcomes in asymptomatic patients undergoing low-risk surgery regardless of age.[3] That said, it is reasonable to obtain a preoperative 12-lead ECG in patients with known cardiac risk factors, a history of coronary artery disease, arrhythmia, cerebral vascular disease, or other significant structural heart disease who are undergoing moderate-risk to high-risk surgical procedures.

A cardiac risk assessment is one of the most important tools for determining a patient's overall cardiac surgical risk. The American College of Surgeons has developed the National Surgical Quality Improvement Program (ACS NSQIP).[12] This calculator is Web based and is available at http://riskcalculator.facs.org/Riskcalculator/. Although the ACS NSQIP has been criticized for not being validated in a group separate from the initial patient population, this calculator can be useful for primary care clinicians because it provides individualized risks for numerous complications and is easy to use.

CHEST RADIOGRAPHY

In a review of clinical guidelines, there is no high-quality evidence (supporting the utility) on the effectiveness of preoperative chest radiography.[13,14] The guidelines agree that routine preoperative chest radiography in asymptomatic, otherwise healthy individuals is not indicated regardless of the planned procedure. They do agree, however, that a baseline radiograph is indicated if a patient has signs or symptoms suggesting a new or unstable cardiopulmonary disease or if a patient is at risk for postoperative pulmonary complications and then only if the results alter the perioperative management.

CONSIDERATIONS FOR ELDERLY PATIENTS

Using age as a criterion for preoperative testing is controversial. There is no doubt that as the age of a patient increases, the more likely the patient is to have abnormal test results: patients aged 70 years or older have an approximately 10% chance of having abnormal levels of serum creatinine, hemoglobin, or glucose and a 75% chance of having at least 1 abnormality on their ECG (and a 50% chance of having a major ECG abnormality).[4] These factors, however, were found not to be predictive of postoperative complications. In contrast, predictive factors for this age group are an American Society of Anesthesiologists physical status classification of at least 3 (indicating severe systemic disease), the risk of the surgical procedure, and a history of congestive heart failure.[15,16]

DISCLOSURE

The authors have nothing to disclose.

REFERENCES

1. Hall MJ, Schwartzman A, Zhang J, et al. Ambulatory surgery data from hospitals and ambulatory surgery centers: United States, 2010. National health statistics reports; no 102. Hyattsville (MD): National Center for Health Statistics; 2017.
2. Society of General Internal Medicine Choosing Wisely recommendations. Available at: https://www.sgim.org/File%20Library/SGIM/Publications/Choosing-Wisely–Preop-Testing–revised-final-web2.pdf. Accessed March 27, 2020.
3. Fleisher LA, Fleischmann Ke, Auerbach AD, et al. American College of Cardiology; American Heart Association. 2014 ACC/AHA guideline on perioperative cardiovascular evaluation and management of patients undergoing noncardiac surgery: a report of the American College of Cardiology/American Heart Association Task Force on practice guidelines. J Am Coll Cardiol 2014;64:e77–137.
4. Hepner DL. The role of testing in the preoperative evaluation. Cleve Clin J Med 2009;76(Suppl 4):S22–7.
5. Feely MA, Collins CS, Daniels PR, et al. Preoperative testing before noncardiac surgery: guidelines and recommendations. Am Fam Physician 2013;87(6):414–8.
6. Bock M, Fritsch G, Hepner D. Preoperative laboratory testing. Anesthesiol Clin 2016;34(1):43–58.
7. Edwards AF, Forest DJ. Preoperative laboratory testing. Anesthesiol Clin 2018;36: 493–507.
8. Roberts JC, Flood VH. Laboratory diagnosis of von Willebrand disease. Int J Lab Hematol 2015;37(Suppl. 1):11–7.
9. Wu WC, Schifftner TL, Henderson WG, et al. Preoperative hematocrit levels and postoperative outcomes in older patients undergoing noncardiac surgery. JAMA 2007;297(22):2481–8.
10. Martin SK, Cifu AS. Routine preoperative laboratory tests for elective surgery. JAMA 2017;318(6):567–8.
11. Umpierrez GE, Isaacs SD, Bazargan N, et al. Hyperglycemia: an independent marker of in-hospital mortality in patients with undiagnosed diabetes. J Clin Endocrinol Metab 2002;87(3):978–82.
12. Bilimoria KY, Liu Y, Paruch JL, et al. Development and evaluation of the universal ACS NSQIP surgical risk calculator: a decision aid and informed consent tool for patients and surgeons. J Am Coll Surg 2013;217(5):833–42.
13. Danielson D, Bjork K, Foreman J, et al. Preoperative evaluation. Inst Clin Syst Improv 2012;10:1–61.
14. National Collaborating Centre for Acute Care (UK). Preoperative tests: the use of routine preoperative tests for elective surgery. London: National Collaborating Centre for Acute Care (UK); 2003 (NICE Clinical Guidelines, No. 3).
15. Dzankic S, Pastor D, Gonzalez C, et al. The prevalence and predictive value of abnormal preoperative laboratory tests in elderly surgical patients. Anesth Analg 2001;93:301–8.
16. Liu LL, Dzankic S, Leung JM. Preoperative electrocardiogram abnormalities do not predict postoperative cardiac complications in geriatric surgical patients. J Am Geriatr Soc 2002;50:1186–91.

Postoperative Ileus

Brennan Bowker, MHS, PA-C, CPAAPA[a],*,
Rebecca Orsulak Calabrese, MHS, PA-C, CPAAPA[b], Emily Barber, MHS, PA-C[c]

KEYWORDS

- Ileus • Postoperative ileus • Paralytic ileus • Surgery

KEY POINTS

- Postoperative ileus (POI) is a transient impairment of bowel function that frequently occurs after major abdominal surgery.
- Although self-limiting, POI is a major contributor to increased length of stay, morbidity, and cost after surgery.
- Enhanced recovery after surgery (ERAS) pathways have been successfully implemented to reduce incidence of POI.
- ERAS pathways focus on early ambulation, reduced opiate use, and other pharmacologic agents that help patients recover more quickly after surgery.

INTRODUCTION

Postoperative ileus (POI) is a transient impairment of bowel function and an often-anticipated complication that occurs in patients who have undergone abdominal or pelvic surgery. POI can occur after some orthopedic surgeries; however, it is most common after intra-abdominal surgery. Although some clinicians think that POI is a normal physiologic response to surgery, it is a major contributor to hospital cost, increased morbidity and mortality, and prolonged hospital course after surgery. Although the pathophysiology of this process remains poorly understood, significant advances have been made in the last decade that have helped ameliorate some of the burden that POI places on the patients and health care systems.

DEFINING POSTOPERATIVE ILEUS

The term ileus originates from the Greek word eileos, which literally means to squeeze or twist.[1] Ironically, the modern use of the word describes a process in which there is cessation or slowed gastrointestinal (GI) transit, the opposite of the word's origin.

[a] Department of Surgery, Emergency and General Surgery, Yale New Haven Hospital, 20 York Street, New Haven, CT 06511, USA; [b] Department of Surgery, Yale New Haven Hospital, 20 York Street, New Haven, CT 06511, USA; [c] Physician Assistant Program, Quinnipiac University, 275 Mt. Carmel Ave, Hamden, CT 06518, USA
* Corresponding author.
E-mail address: Brennan.bowker@quinnipiac.edu

Physician Assist Clin 6 (2021) 215–227
https://doi.org/10.1016/j.cpha.2020.12.001
2405-7991/21/© 2020 Elsevier Inc. All rights reserved.
physicianassistant.theclinics.com

Although many agree on this misnomer, there still is no generalized consensus for the definition of POI, despite Kehlet and colleagues[2] in 2005 suggesting that a common definition was needed. In 2013, Vather and colleagues[3] performed a systematic review of 52 studies and, from that, developed recommendations for the definition of POI, prolonged POI (PPOI), and recurrent POI (**Table 1**). From this, he defined POI as the time from surgery until the patient has passed flatus or stool and has tolerated a diet, noting that these events should occur on or before postoperative day 4.[3] Van Bree and colleagues[4] corroborated Kehlet and colleagues'[2] definitions in 2014, but there still remains a lack of consensus on the time frame for which POI and PPOI should be defined. Most studies suggest a period between 3 and 7 days for POI,[3,5–9] although the time at which POI transitions to PPOI has not been well delineated[10]; a 2015 study by Moghadamyeghaneh and colleagues[6] set a time frame of no return of bowel function within 7 days of surgery, and this seems to be largely agreed on.

INCIDENCE OF POSTOPERATIVE ILEUS AFTER SURGERY

Given the ambiguity of the definition, it is difficult both to study this condition and to determine the true incidence of POI; rates for colorectal surgery vary between 10% and 30%.[3,5–9,11,12] Similarly, PPOI rates are not well defined but incidences have been reported between 12.7%[6] and 15.9%.[10] Despite the variability, even the rates on the lower end of the spectrum are significant. Curiously, rates of POI after gastric and pancreatic procedures seem to be lower, with incidences ranging between 8% and 13%,[13] although some studies show a higher risk of prolonged ileus with rates near 20%.[14] In addition, POI has been observed in patients undergoing orthopedic procedures such as total knee and total hip arthroplasty. Unlike their intra-abdominal counterparts, total joint arthroplasty (TJA) is low risk for POI development, with rates less than 1%.[15] POI after spine surgery is much more common than after TJA, but, at an incidence of about 7%, rates are still much lower than intra-abdominal interventions.[16]

Table 1
Vather's classification of postoperative ileus[7]

	Criteria	Time
POI	• Passage of flatus or stool • Tolerance of a diet (by mouth)	Both criteria must be met on or before POD 4
Prolonged POI	• Nausea or vomiting • Inability to tolerate PO over the prior 24 h • Absence of flatus over the prior 24 h • Abdominal distention • Radiologic confirmation	Two or more of the 5 criteria met on or after POD 4 without prior resolution of a POI
Recurrent POI	• Nausea or vomiting • Inability to tolerate PO over the prior 24 h • Absence of flatus over the prior 24 h • Abdominal distention • Radiologic confirmation	Two or more of the 5 criteria met after resolution of a prior POI

Abbreviations: PO, per os; POD, postoperative day.

PATHOPHYSIOLOGY OF THE POSTOPERATIVE ILEUS

The pathophysiology by which POI occurs is an extremely complex interplay between autonomic and hormonal mechanisms and is thought to occur in 3 distinct phases: neurologic phase, inflammatory phase, and resolution/vagal activation phase. During the neurologic phase, presynaptic noradrenergic B receptors are activated by the anesthetic and the surgical incision.[17] It is then alleged that these receptors act on the enteric nervous system, resulting in instability of the intestinal mucosal barrier secondary to glial cell impairment.[18] In addition, this inflammation increases messenger RNA (mRNA) synthesis of inducible nitric oxide synthase (iNOS), which then releases nitrogen monoxide and, as a result, then activates cyclooxygenase-2 (COX2) inflammation.[19–22]

The second phase begins as the first phase ends and is characterized by increasing inflammation in the intestinal wall. Anatomically, the muscularis externa is inhabited by a dense network of macrophages, which are then activated by handling of the intestine during surgery.[23] This cascade is mostly seen after the third hour of surgery and is not observed in strictly laparoscopic procedures. Also during this phase, T1 helper lymphocytes are activated by interleukin; these cells then migrate to nonmanipulated areas and induce the inflammatory cascade there. Bacterial translocation is also noted, which can further propagate the inflammatory response.[24]

In addition, the resolution of this process is mediated by increased vagal tone, which then reduces the incited inflammatory cascade. Acetylcholine is released, thereby activating the α7-nAcHr (alpha 7 nicotinic acetylcholinase receptor) on monocytes and macrophages. This activation consequently reduces inflammation.[25]

It is also important to note the potential role of potassium in propagation of POI. Basic science has shown that potassium partakes in depolarization of smooth muscle membranes, which then allows voltage-dependent calcium channels to open, allowing an influx of calcium and subsequent smooth muscle contraction. A link between hypokalemia and POI was first noted in a 1970 by Lowman[26] when he observed that ileus resolved with the correction of hypokalemia. A more recent cohort study by Sanger and Tuladhar[27] noted similar results.

In addition to hypokalemia, opiate use is also highly implicated in gut dysmotility and ileus formation after surgery. Opiates stimulate the μ-opioid receptors in the bowel wall,[28] which subsequently leads to decreased secretions and overall an inhibitory effect on peristalsis.[29] Studies have shown that only a quarter of the dose required for adequate analgesia after surgery results in significant inhibition of peristalsis,[30,31] which suggests that opioid usage is a major contributor to POI. However, this effect is further amplified in individuals with opioid tolerance because intestinal receptors do not seem to develop the same tolerance,[28] thereby worsening the effect after surgery.

TYPES OF POSTOPERATIVE ILEUS

Recovery of GI motility is not equal across the entire GI tract. Typically, the small intestine recovers first, often within 24 hours, which is then followed by the stomach (48 hours), and lastly the large intestine (3–5 days).[32] With this knowledge, a panel of experts from the Postoperative Ileus Management Council have determined there to be 3 different classifications of POI based on the afflicted portion of the GI tract (**Table 2**). Type I is also referred to as panintestinal and involves both upper and lower portions of the GI tract. Patients afflicted by type I POI often manifest early after surgery with obstipation, and unrelenting nausea and vomiting. These patients often require nasogastric decompression for symptomatic relief. Type II POI affects only

Table 2
Classification of postoperative ileus by type[33]

	Location	Symptoms	Treatment
Type I	Panintestinal	Persistent nausea Persistent vomiting No flatus or stool	Symptomatic NG tube
Type II	Upper GI tract	Persistent nausea Persistent vomiting ± Distention May have flatus or stool despite nausea	Symptomatic NG tube Rule out mechanical obstruction
Type III	Lower GI tract	No flatus or stool Tolerates diet No nausea/vomiting	Watchful waiting

Abbreviation: NG, nasogastric.

the upper GI tract. Similar to patients with type I POI, these patients experience persistent nausea and vomiting but also may or may not have abdominal distention. Clinically, type II POI presents in a fashion almost indistinguishable from small bowel obstruction and, therefore, further investigation may be warranted. Type III POI occurs in the lower GI tract only and represents a small portion of POI cases. Patients with type III POI are typically obstipated but without the nausea, vomiting, and distention often seen with types I and II. These patients also, typically, tolerate a diet by mouth several days before the return of flatus or bowel movements.[33]

RISK FACTORS FOR DEVELOPING POSTOPERATIVE ILEUS AFTER INTRA-ABDOMINAL SURGERY

Several risk factors for the development of POI and PPOI have been identified. These risk factors include male sex, open procedure, laparoscopy converted to open, resection of the rectum, and mobilization of the splenic flexure.[10] Other studies have also identified preoperative and postoperative narcotic use, advanced age, respiratory comorbidities such as chronic obstructive pulmonary disease, duration of surgery, operative difficulty (and subsequent increased handling of the intestine), and volume crystalloid administration as risk factors in POI formation.[3,5,7–10,34] In addition, several studies have also delineated that patients with a preoperative American Society of Anesthesiologists (ASA) score of III or greater are at higher risk not only of POI but also for its subsequent complications.[35,36] Emergency surgery, delayed mobilization, and use of parenteral nutrition have also all been found to be contributors to POI.[6,37,38]

DIAGNOSIS

POI is a clinical diagnosis; abdominal distension, tenderness, and the absence of normal bowel sounds have been identified as the most relevant clinical signs,[39] although recent studies have shown a lack of association between bowel sounds and return of bowel function.[40] There are no evidence-based guidelines that support the use of an imaging modality in the diagnosis of POI. Imaging is used to rule out other common postoperative complications, because there is significant overlap in clinical presentation.[39] POI and mechanical intestinal obstruction can present in a similar fashion. Furthermore, PPOI has been associated with other postoperative complications, such as anastomotic leak and intra-abdominal infections; therefore, underlying processes must be considered before accepting the process to be simply physiologic.[6]

Although plain abdominal radiographs are often the initial imaging study in the work-up of these clinical symptoms (**Fig. 1**),[41] computed tomography (CT) is the best diagnostic tool to rule out other postoperative complications.[42] CT scan is the best imaging modality if small bowel obstruction (SBO) is suspected,[43] and is more sensitive and specific than plain radiographs in distinguishing between SBO and POI.[44] CT scan in mechanical obstruction can show proximal bowel dilatation, a discrete transition zone, and fully or partially collapsed distal bowel, whereas POI is radiologically identified by diffuse small and large bowel dilatation without a distinct transition zone.[44,45]

DIFFERENTIAL DIAGNOSIS: NOT ALL ILEUSES ARE CREATED EQUALLY

Although some form of surgical intervention is required to make the diagnosis of POI, an ileus can occur for other reasons even after surgical intervention. For example, urine is extremely irritating to the intestine and has been linked to ileus development after robotic cystectomy; in cases such as this, the ileus is caused not by the mechanisms previously described but by an anastomotic failure, for instance, causing urine leak.[46] Blood and enteric contents are also extremely irritating and can cause paralytic ileus via alternative mechanisms. It is important to consider leak in patients who develop an ileus when you would have otherwise expected them not to or when patients fail to progress as expected after surgery. In addition, medications such as calcium channel blockers[47] and magnesium[48] (at increased levels) have been known to cause ileus, as have less common conditions such as Guillain-Barré syndrome,[49] pheochromocytoma,[50] strongyloidiasis infection,[51] and hypothyroidism.[52]

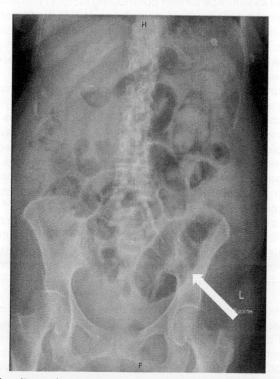

Fig. 1. Abdominal radiograph. Nonspecific dilated small bowel loops (*arrows*) without a definitive transition point consistent with POI.

In addition to functional causes of dysmotility, mechanical causes of obstruction should be kept on the differential, even after surgery. Potential postoperative bowel obstruction can occur from internal hernia, abdominal wall hernia, intussusception, foreign body (or retained foreign body), gallstones, volvulus, or stool impaction. In addition, colonic pseudo-obstruction (Ogilvie syndrome) should also be kept on the differential. Although none of these are particularly common immediately after surgery, these diagnoses should be ruled out in patients who fail to progress.

TREATMENT AND PREVENTION OF POSTOPERATIVE ILEUS

All patients with POI should be treated supportively with appropriate fluid balance and electrolyte correction. Antiemetics should be used to reduce episodes of emesis and consequent potential risk for aspiration. Nasogastric tube decompression may be required in patients with repeated episodes of emesis; however, this has been correlated with longer hospitalizations and poorer patient satisfaction scores. Supplemental total parenteral nutrition should be considered for patients who are unable to tolerate liquids or solid food by mouth for greater than 7 days.

Aside from supportive therapy, much of the treatment of POI lies in prevention. Prevention of POI is multifactorial, including pharmacologic and nonpharmacologic modalities, and spans across the entire perioperative period. Early ambulation,[37] early resumption of diet,[38] coffee,[53] and the Japanese herb dai-kenchu-to[54,55] have all been explored as potential prevention strategies for POI prevention. However, no single modality has been identified to prevent the development of POI.

Opioids are well known to be a major contributing factor in the development of POI. Opiate pain medications bind to the μ-opioid receptors in the GI tract, slowing down bowel motility and GI recovery.[56] Using adjuvant pain medication, such as acetaminophen, ketorolac, ibuprofen, and gabapentin, can help decrease opioid requirements for adequate pain control. Regional blocks and epidural anesthesia, when appropriate, can also assist in limiting narcotic effect on the GI tract.

Regional anesthetic infiltration in the form of transversus abdominus plane (TAP) blocks are often used as a part of the enhanced recovery pathways and have been proved to decrease need for narcotic use in the early postoperative phase. A recent meta-analysis found that TAP blocks significantly decrease pain with coughing and moving after colorectal surgery.[57] This effect then allows patients to ambulate comfortably immediately after surgery, which may have a role in decreasing ileus.

Nonsteroidal antiinflammatory drugs (NSAIDs) can be used either singularly or in conjunction with regional anesthetics to target the COX2-mediated inflammatory cascade that occurs during the second phase of ileus formation.[58] However, some colorectal surgeons cautiously use NSAIDs because of their potential implication in anastomotic dehiscence.[59,60] Other strategies that have been thought to help prevent POI include the use of epidural anesthesia, although data are mixed on the efficacy of this strategy in colorectal surgery,[61,62] as well as using laparoscopic approaches (when possible) because this has been shown to decrease ileus by 30% in some cohorts.[63]

In addition to minimizing narcotic use and using multimodal pain control, protocols such as enhanced recovery after surgery (ERAS), which encompasses a multitude of evidence-based practices,[56] have collectively been shown to reduce the incidence of POI when adhered to. Consequently, ERAS has also been found to decrease length of stay and overall cost of care. Patients without POI recover faster and are more satisfied with their care. ERAS begins in the preoperative setting with preoperative counseling. Patients are educated by their surgical and anesthesia teams about POI and the measures they can take to reduce their risk. When clinically appropriate, patients are instructed to increase preoperative sweetened liquids, consume immunonutrition agents if preoperative malnutrition is of concern, and reduce preoperative fasting (to allow for solid intake within 6 hours before surgery and clear liquids up to 2 hours before surgery). Providers should avoid prescribing any bowel preparation if possible, unless midrectal or low-rectal resections are being performed. Intraoperatively, the anesthesia team should make every effort to avoid postoperative nausea. Intravenous fluids should be limited and used judiciously based on length of surgery. Fluids should be warmed and warming blankets used in an attempt to maintain normothermia throughout the procedure. From a surgical perspective, laparoscopic surgery is preferred to open when appropriate. If a nasogastric tube is used intraoperatively, it should be removed before the patient emerges from anesthesia.[64]

Postoperatively, patients on ERAS protocols have several guidelines to reduce their risk of POI. Continued restrictive use of intravenous fluid, early urinary catheter removal, early mobilization, multimodal pain control (with a focus on minimizing narcotics), and incentive spirometry use are all included in ERAS. Early oral intake is also encouraged and most patients can be started on clear liquids within 6 hours of the procedure. Medications or therapies that promote bowel motility, such as magnesium citrate or chewing gum, are also often used.[64]

On review of an observational prospective single-center study conducted with 131 patients, it was shown that improved outcomes were directly related to how strictly the ERAS guidelines were adhered to. When compliance with ERAS was less than 85%, 46.5% of patients developed a POI, compared with 26.7% when compliance with ERAS was more than 85%. During this study, it was noted that the postoperative components of ERAS were the most difficult for patients and providers to adhere to. Adherence to the protocol may be improved with increased education of health care staff caring for the patients and performing audits to track compliance.[64]

Gum chewing, a component of ERAS, is considered a preventive measure on its own. Chewing gum is inexpensive, safe, and is known to stimulate bowel motility. By allowing patients to chew gum, the process of mastication is mimicked, therefore stimulating vagal tone. Although a low-risk intervention, the data showing the efficacy of gum chewing are mixed and what positive data do exist come from small cohorts. A prospective randomized trial of 64 patients undergoing elective colorectal surgery noted that patients who chewed gum had less nausea, fewer episodes of emesis, reduced incidence of POI, and decreased length of hospital stay.[65] The use of nicotine gum has also been examined because the nicotine provides some antiinflammatory effect, thus targeting phase 2.[66]

In addition, several pharmacologic agents have been studied in the prevention and treatment of POI. Medications thought to stimulate the GI tract, such as erythromycin, metoclopramide, vasopressin, and β-blockers, were all found to be ineffective in stimulating bowel motility in patients with POI. Some studies have revealed that mosapride, a serotonin receptor agonist, significantly improved the time until return of bowel function.[67]

Alvimopan, a highly selective, peripheral μ-opioid receptor antagonist, was approved by the US Food and Drug Administration (FDA) in 2008 for use in certain patients for the prevention of POI. Alvimopan does not easily cross the blood-brain barrier and therefore is able to block the effects of opiates on the GI tract with little effect on postoperative analgesia control. Its use has been shown to be favorable in reducing POI. A meta-analysis of 9 studies published between 2001 and 2014 examined the efficacy of different dosing regimens of alvimopan in 4075 patients who had undergone bowel resection, radical total abdominal hysterectomy, simple total abdominal hysterectomy, or radical cystectomy. When comparing 6-mg dosing, 12-mg dosing, and placebos, both doses significantly reduced the need for nasogastric tube reinsertion and constipation with no effect on postoperative pain control. However, the 12-mg dose was superior in improving the time of bowel function return, decreasing hospital length of stay, and reducing nausea, vomiting, and abdominal distention, and had no effect on postoperative pain control. At present, the FDA recommends the 12-mg dose; however, its use is highly controlled: it is restricted to inpatients and limited to 15 doses. Patients are often prescribed the first dose 2 hours before surgery in the preoperative holding area and continue postoperatively until return of bowel function or discharge home, often whichever comes first.[56]

Although generally considered safe and well tolerated, some adverse cardiovascular events have been noted in patients taking alvimopan. Tachycardia and myocardial infarction have occurred in some patients taking lower doses for nononcologic opioid-induced constipation. Other studies reveal similar rates of cardiovascular events in alvimopan and placebo groups.[56] Despite this, alvimopan is generally thought to be safe and is frequently used in many facilities.

Prucalopride is a highly selective, high-affinity 5-HT$_4$ (serotonin type 4) receptor agonist that has been shown to promote GI tract motility in patients with functional constipation refractory to diet modifications and laxative use. The use of prucalopride for POI has been studied in rats, mice, and humans; all of these studies revealed potential but with limitations, because significant diarrhea and headache were reported. It currently is not a recommended treatment modality for POI; however, this could change with ongoing research.[68]

Gastrografin is a hyperosmolar contrast medium used in certain radiographic diagnostic studies performed for POI or SBO symptoms. Because of its hyperosmolar nature, it can reduce bowel edema and improves intestinal transit by mobilizing extracellular fluid into the GI lumen. A 2-arm, parallel, 1:1 double-blinded, randomized control trial comparing Gastrografin with placebo was not able to show any statistically significant differences in the 2 groups. However, slight differences in favor of Gastrografin were revealed, including reduced duration of nasogastric decompression, improved time to return of bowel function or toleration of oral intake after POI, and overall decreased length of hospitalization.[69]

Simethicone, is a safe, affordable, and easily accessible oral medication that joins gas bubbles in the GI tract to expedite their movement. It has been previously studied in patients who have undergone gynecologic surgery and, in those randomized controlled trials, its use has led to less severe gas pains, earlier return of bowel function, and overall reduced rates of POI. A multicenter, double-blinded, randomized controlled study of 118 patients undergoing colorectal surgery was performed to compare patients receiving simethicone with those in a placebo group. Although this study revealed no statistically significant reduction in time to return of bowel function, it was limited by a small sample size and several missed doses of medication. Given its safety profile, simethicone can be considered as an adjuvant therapy in POI.[70]

ECONOMIC IMPACT

Worldwide, POI and PPOI are huge financial encumbrances on health care systems. Not only do these conditions contribute to longer lengths of stay and higher rates of complication, they also nearly double the cost of an inpatient hospital stay. A recent study in New Zealand found that patients with PPOI had a 71% increase in hospital cost compared with patients without PPOI, which amounts to an average of US$17,332.42 increase in cost.[71] An American study published in 2015 examined hospital cost in patients undergoing open and laparoscopic colectomy as well as patients undergoing open and laparoscopic cholecystectomy. Akin to Mao and colleagues,[71] this study found a similarly large increase in cost, with an average hospital cost of a patient with a POI being $21,046 compared with the cost of a patient without an ileus of $10,945. Thirty-day readmission rates were also examined and found to be statistically significant ($P<.0001$) in all patients who developed POI; this, of course, also contributes to higher health care costs.[72] Although there are few recent data, POI and PPOI are estimated to cost the US health care system $1.46 billion dollars annually.[73] Given the extreme cost to the health care system, there is a strong need to continue to study and understand this complication with the hopes that ongoing advances will be able to mitigate this costly process.

SUMMARY

POI is an extremely physiologically complex and costly complication that can occur after any surgery but is most common after intra-abdominal and pelvic interventions. Characterized by nausea, vomiting, and the overall failure of return of bowel function, POI increases patient discomfort, length of stay, morbidity and mortality, and overall strain on the health care system. In the last decade, researchers have learned more about the pathophysiology and risk factors of POI, which has led to the development of medications such as alvimopan and enhanced recovery pathways, which seem to have improved outcomes slightly. A lot is still unknown about this process, and further research is needed to help in reducing the number of cases and subsequent cost of the disease.

CLINICS CARE POINTS

- POI is a transient impairment of bowel function that frequently occurs after major abdominal surgery.
- Although self-limiting, POI is a major contributor to increased length of stay, morbidity, and cost after surgery.
- ERAS pathways have been successfully implemented to reduce incidence of POI.
- ERAS pathways focus on early ambulation, reduced opiate use, and other pharmacologic agents that help patients recover more quickly after surgery.
- Using local analgesics such as regional nerve blocks and pharmacologic agents such as alvimopan are particularly helpful in reducing ileus after surgery.
- If patients do go on to develop POI, little can be done to hasten its occurrence. In these situations, it is best to provide optimal supportive care to the patient, including adequate resuscitation and electrolyte balance.

DISCLOSURE

The authors have nothing to disclose.

REFERENCES

1. Phipps M, Bush JA, Buhrow D, et al. Ileus development in the trauma/surgical intensive care unit: a process improvement evaluation. Dimens Crit Care Nurs 2011;30(3):164.

2. Kehlet H, Williamson R, Buchler MW, et al. A survey of perceptions and attitudes among European surgeons toward the clinical impact and management of postoperative ileus. Colorectal Dis 2005;7:245–50.
3. Vather R, Trivedi S, Bissett I. Defining postoperative ileus: results of a systematic review and global survey. J Gastrointest Surg 2013;17:962–72.
4. Van Bree SHW, Bemelman WA, Hollmann MW, et al. Identification of clinical outcome measures for recovery of gastrointestinal motility in postoperative ileus. Ann Surg 2014;259:708–14.
5. Chapuis PH, Bokey L, Keshava A, et al. Risk factors for prolonged ileus after resection of colorectal cancer: an observational study of 2400 consecutive patients. Ann Surg 2014;257:909–15.
6. Moghadamyeghaneh Z, Hwang GS, Hanna MH, et al. Risk factors for prolonged ileus following colon surgery. Surg Endosc 2016;30:603–9.
7. Vather R, Josephson R, Jaung R, et al. Development of a risk stratification system for the occurrence of prolonged postoperative ileus after colorectal surgery: a prospective risk factor analysis. Surgery 2015;157:764–73.
8. Artinyan A, Nunoo-Mensah JW, Balasubramaniam S, et al. Prolonged postoperative ileus-definition, risk factors, and predictors after surgery. World J Surg 2008; 32:1495–500.
9. Millan M, Biondo S, Fraccalvieri D, et al. Risk factors for prolonged postoperative ileus after colorectal cancer surgery. World J Surg 2012;36:179–85.
10. Wolthuis AM, Bislenghi G, Lambrecht M, et al. Preoperative risk factors for prolonged postoperative ileus after colon resection. Int J Colorectal Dis 2017;32: 883–90.
11. Svatek RS, Fisher MB, Williams MB, et al. Age and body mass index are independent risk factors for the development of postoperative paralytic ileus after radical cystectomy. Urology 2010;76:1419–24.
12. Kim MJ, Min GE, Yoo KH, et al. Risk factors for postoperative ileus after urologic laparoscopic surgery. J Korean Surg Soc 2011;17:962–72.
13. Shah J, Shah DR, Brown E, et al. Negligible effect of perioperative epidural analgesia among patients undergoing elective gastric and pancreatic resections. J Gastrointest Surg 2013;17:660–7.
14. Liang WQ, Zhang KC, Cui JX, et al. Nomogram to predict prolonged postoperative ileus after gastrectomy in gastric cancer. World J Gastroenterol 2019;25(38): 5838–49.
15. Klasan A, Amic F, Dworschak P, et al. Risk factors for ileus after hip and knee arthroplasty. Int J Colorectal Dis 2019;34:261–7.
16. Durand WM, Ruddell JH, Eltorai AEM, et al. Ileus following adult spinal deformity surgery. World Neurosurg 2018;116:e806–13.
17. Goetz B, Benhaqi P, Muller MH, et al. Changes in beta adrenergic neurotransmission during postoperative ileus in rat circular jejunal muscle. Neurogastroenterol Motil 2013;25:e154–84.
18. Neunlist M, Rolli-Derkinderen M, Latorre R, et al. Enteric glial cells: recent developments and future directions. Gastroenterology 2014;147:1230–7.
19. Kreiss C, Birder LA, Kiss S, et al. COX-2 dependent inflammation increases spinal fos expression during rodent postoperative ileus. Gut 2003;52:527–34.
20. Yanagida H, Sanders KM, Ward SM. Inactivation of inducible nitric oxide synthase protects intestinal pacemaker cells from postoperative damage. J Physiol 2007;582:755–65.
21. Turler A, Kalff JC, Moore BA, et al. Leukocyte-derived inducible nitric oxide synthase mediates murine postoperative ileus. Ann Surg 2006;244:220–9.

22. Schwarz NT, Beer-Stolz D, Simmons RL, et al. Pathogenesis of paralytic ileus: Intestinal manipulation opens a transient pathway between the intestinal lumen and the leukocytic infiltrate of the jejunal muscularis. Ann Surg 2002;235:31–40.

23. Kalff JC, Schraut WH, Simmons RL, et al. Surgical manipulation of the gut elicits an intestinal muscularis inflammatory response resulting in postsurgical ileus. Ann Surg 1998;228:652–63.

24. The FO, Bennik RJ, Ankum WM, et al. Intestinal handling induced mast cell activation and inflammation in human postoperative ileus. Gut 2008;57:33–40.

25. Tsuchida Y, Hatao F, Fujisawa M, et al. Neuronal stimulation with 5-hydroxytryptamine 4 receptor induces anti-inflammatory actions via alpha-7nACh receptors on muscularis macrophages associated with postoperative ileus. Gut 2011;60: 638–47.

26. Lowman RM. The potassium depletion states and postoperative ileus. The role of the potassium ion. Radiology 1971;98:691–4.

27. Sanger GJ, Tuladhar BR. The role of endogenous opioids in the control of gastrointestinal motility: predictions from in vitro modeling. Neurogastroenterol Motil 2004;16(Suppl. 2):38–45.

28. Holte K, Kehlet H. Postoperative ileus: progress towards effective management. Drugs 2002;62:2603–15.

29. Bauer AJ, Boeckxstaens GE. Mechanisms of postoperative ileus. Neurogastroenterol Motil 2004;16(Suppl 2):54–60.

30. Holte K, Kehlet H. Postoperative ileus: a preventable event. Br J Surg 2000;87: 1480–93.

31. Sternini C, Patierno S, Selmer IS, et al. The opioid system in the gastrointestinal tract. Neurogastroenterol Motil 2004;16(Suppl 2):3–16.

32. Livingston EH, Passaro EP. Postoperative ileus. Dig Dis Sci 1990;35:121–32.

33. Delaney C, Kehlet H, Senagore A, et al. Postoperative ileus: profiles, risk factors, and definitions-a framework for optimizing surgical outcomes in patients undergoing major abdominal colorectal surgery. In: Bosker G, editor. Clinical consensus update in general surgery. Roswell (GA): Pharmatecture, LLC; 2006. p. 1–26.

34. Kronberg U, Kiran RP, Soliman MSM, et al. A characterization of factors determining postoperative ileus after laparoscopic colectomy enables the generation of a novel predictive score. Ann Surg 2011;253(1):78–81.

35. Grass F, Slieker J, Jurt J. Postoperative ileus in an enhanced recovery pathway: a retrospective cohort study. Int J Colorectal Dis 2017;32:675–81.

36. Vlug MS, Bartels SA, Wind J, et al. Which fast track elements predict early recovery after colon cancer surgery? Colorectal Dis 2012;14(8):1001–8.

37. Bragg D, El-Sharkawy AM, Psaltis E, et al. Postoperative ileus: recent developments in pathophysiology and management. Clin Nutr 2015;34:367–76.

38. Boelens PG, Heesakkers FF, Luyer MD, et al. Reduction of postoperative ileus by early enteral nutrition in patients undergoing major rectal surgery: prospective, randomized, controlled trial. Ann Surg 2014;259:649–55.

39. Gero D, Gié O, Hübner M, et al. Postoperative ileus: in search of an international consensus on definition, diagnosis, and treatment. Langenbecks Arch Surg 2017;402:149–58.

40. Read TE, Brozovich M, Andujar JE, et al. Bowel sounds are not associated with flatus, bowel movement, or tolerance of oral intake in patients after major abdominal surgery. Dis Colon Rectum 2017;60:608–13.

41. Allen AM, Antosh DD, Grimes CL, et al. Management of ileus and small-bowel obstruction following benign gynecologic surgery. Int J Gynecol Obstet 2013; 121(1):56–9.
42. Wu Z, Boersema GSA, Dereci A, et al. Clinical endpoint, early detection, and differential diagnosis of postoperative ileus: a systematic review of the literature. Eur Surg Res 2015;54:127–38.
43. Ten Broek RPG, Krielen P, Di Saverio S, et al. Bologna guidelines for diagnosis and management of adhesive small bowel obstruction (ASBO): 2017 update of the evidence-based guidelines from the world society of emergency surgery ASBO working group. World J Emerg Surg 2018;13:24.
44. Frager DH, Baer JW, Rothpearl A, et al. Distinction between postoperative ileus and mechanical small-bowel obstruction: value of CT compared with clinical and other radiographic findings. Am J Roentgenol 1995;164:891–4.
45. Frager D, Medwid SW, Baer JW, et al. CT of small-bowel obstruction: value in establishing the diagnosis and determining the degree and cause. Am J Roentgenol 1994;162(1):37–41.
46. Ozdemir AT, Altinova S, Koyuncu H, et al. The incidence of postoperative ileus in patients who underwent robotic assisted radical prostatectomy. Cent European J Urol 2014;67(1):19–24.
47. Wright S, Ali M, Robinson A, et al. Paralytic ileus associated with use of diltiazem. Am J Health Syst Pharm 2011;68(15):1426–9.
48. Al-Shoha M, Klair JS, Girotra M, et al. Magnesium toxicity-induced ileus in a postpartum patient treated for preeclampsia with magnesium sulfate. ACG Case Rep J 2015;2(4):227–9.
49. Nowe T, Huttemann K, Engelhorn T, et al. Paralytic ileus as a presenting symptom of Guillain-Barre syndrome. J Neurol 2008;255:756–7.
50. Noguchi M, Taniya T, Ueno K, et al. A case of pheochromocytoma with severe paralytic ileus. Jpn J Surg 1990;20:448–50.
51. Yoshida H, Endo H, Tanaka S, et al. Recurrent paralytic ileus associated with strongyloidiasis in a patient with systemic lupus erythematosus. Mod Rheumatol 2006;16:44–7.
52. Rodrigo C, Gamakaranage CSSSK, Epa DS, et al. Hypothyroidism causing paralytic ileus and acute kidney injury: case report. Thyroid Res 2011;4(7):4–7.
53. Muller SA, Rahbari NN, Schneider F, et al. Randomized clinical trial on the effect of coffee on postoperative ileus following elective colectomy. Br J Surg 2012;99: 1530–8.
54. Yaegashi M, Otsuka K, Itabashi T, et al. Daikenchuto stimulates colonic motility after laparoscopic-assisted colectomy. Hepatogastroenterology 2014;61:85–9.
55. Akamaru Y, Takahashi T, Nishida T, et al. Effects of daikenchuto, a Japanese herb, on intestinal motility after total gastrectomy: a prospective randomized trial. J Gastrointest Surg 2015;19:467–72.
56. Xu LL, Zhou XQ, Yi PS, et al. Alvimopan combined with enhanced recovery strategy for managing postoperative ileus after open abdominal surgery: a systematic review and meta-analysis. J Surg Res 2016;203:211–21.
57. Peltrini R, Cantoni V, Green R, et al. Efficacy of transversus abdominis plane (TAP) block in colorectal surgery: a systematic review and meta-analysis. Tech Coloproctol 2020;24(8):787–802.
58. Sim R, Cheong DM, Wong KS, et al. Prospective randomized, double-blind, placebo-controlled study of pre and postoperative administration of a COX-2-specific inhibitor as opioid-sparing analgesia in major colorectal surgery. Colorectal Dis 2007;9:51–60.

59. Schlachta CM, Burpee SE, Fernandez C, et al. Optimizing recovery after laparoscopic colon surgery (ORAL-CS): effect of intravenous ketorolac on length of hospital stay. Surg Endosc 2007;21:2212–9.

60. Holte K, Andersen J, Jakobsen DH, et al. Cyclo-oxygenase 2 inhibitors and the risk of anastomotic leakage after fast-track colon surgery. Br J Surg 2009;96: 650–4.

61. Halabi WJ, Kang CY, Nguyen VQ, et al. Epidural analgesia in laparoscopic colorectal surgery: a nationwide analysis of use and outcomes. JAMA Surg 2014;149: 130–6.

62. Hubner M, Blanc C, Roulin D, et al. Randomized clinical trial on epidural versus patient-controlled analgesia for laparoscopic colorectal surgery within an enhanced recovery pathway. Ann Surg 2015;261:648–53.

63. Gervaz P, Inan I, Perneger T, et al. A prospective, randomized, single-blind comparison of laparoscopic versus open sigmoid colectomy for diverticulitis. Ann Surg 2010;252:3–8.

64. Barbieux J, Hamy A, Talbot MF, et al. Does enhanced recovery reduce postoperative ileus after colorectal surgery. J Visc Surg 2017;154:79–85.

65. Vergara-Fernandez O, Gonzalez-Vargas AP, Castellanos-Juarez JC, et al. Usefulness of gum chewing to decrease postoperative ileus in colorectal surgery wit primary anastomosis: a randomized controlled trial. Rev Invest Clin 2016;68: 314–8.

66. Wu Z, Boersema GSA, Jeekel J, et al. Nicotine gum chewing: a novel strategy to shorten duration of postoperative ileus via vagus nerve activation. Med Hypotheses 2014;83:352–4.

67. Drake TM, Ward AE. Pharmacological management to prevent ileus in major abdominal surgery: a systematic review and meta-analysis. J Gastrointest Surg 2016;20(6):1253–64.

68. Smart C, Malik K. Prucalopride for the treatment of ileus. Expert Opin Investig Drugs 2017;26(4):489–93.

69. Biondo S, Miquel J, Espin-Basany E, et al. A double-blinded randomized clinical study on the therapeutic effect of Gastrografin in prolonged postoperative ileus after elective colorectal surgery. World J Surg 2016;40(1):206–14.

70. Springer J, Elkheir S, Eskicioglu C, et al. The effect of simethicone on postoperative ileus in patients undergoing colorectal surgery (SPOT), a randomized controlled trial. Int J Surg 2018;65:141–7.

71. Mao H, Milne TGE, O'Grady G, et al. Prolonged postoperative ileus significantly increases the cost of inpatient stay for patients undergoing elective colorectal surgery: results of a multivariate analysis of prospective data at a single institution. Dis Colon Rectum 2019;62(5):631–7.

72. Gan TJ, Robinson SB, Oderda GM, et al. Impact of postsurgical opioid use and ileus on economic outcomes in gastrointestinal surgeries. Curr Med Res Opin 2015;31(4):677–86.

73. Brady JT, Dosokey EM, Crawshaw BP, et al. The use of alvimopan for postoperative ileus in small and large bowel resections. Expert Rev Gastroenterol Hepatol 2015;9:1351–8.

Periprosthetic Joint Infections of the Hip and Knee

A Review of Preoperative Diagnosis and Treatment Options

Kristi A. Collins, MS, PA-C

KEYWORDS

- Periprosthetic joint infection • Total joint arthroplasty • Total hip arthroplasty
- Total knee arthroplasty

KEY POINTS

- Periprosthetic joint infection can be characterized as acute postoperative, acute hematogenous, or chronic based on the duration of symptoms and time since the index procedure.
- Common presenting symptoms include persistent wound drainage, joint effusion, fever, acute/chronic joint pain, persistent stiffness, or decreased range of motion.
- The preoperative workup includes serum erythrocyte sedimentation rate and C-reactive protein, serum D-dimer, synovial fluid culture, cell count and differential, leukocyte esterase, alpha-defensin, and synovial fluid erythrocyte sedimentation rate.
- Gram-positive organisms are commonly implicated, including *Staphylococcus aureus*, coagulase-negative *Staphylococci*, and *Enterococi* and *Streptococi* spp.; polymicrobial and culture-negative infections also occur.
- Depending on chronicity of the infection, treatment may include debridement, antibiotics, irrigation and retention of implants, and single-stage or 2-stage revision.

INTRODUCTION

Total joint arthroplasties (TJA) are common orthopedic procedures. Periprosthetic joint infection (PJI), although relatively infrequent, is a disastrous complication of total hip and knee arthroplasty. Combined rates of infection for primary and revision arthroplasty are around 1%, with infection rates being significantly higher for revision arthroplasties than primary arthroplasties.[1–5] For affected patients, PJI carries significant morbidity and mortality risk. Treatment of PJI, as compared with revision arthroplasty

Physician Assistant Program, Franklin Pierce University, 24 Airport Road, Suite 19, West Lebanon, NH 03784, USA
E-mail address: collinskr@franklinpierce.edu

Physician Assist Clin 6 (2021) 229–238
https://doi.org/10.1016/j.cpha.2020.11.006
2405-7991/21/© 2020 Elsevier Inc. All rights reserved.

for other causes, has been associated with longer hospital stays, higher rates of medical complications, an increased need for transfusion, higher readmission rates, and more discharges to locations other than home.[6] In addition, the mortality risk for patients undergoing surgical treatment of PJI is up to 5 times greater than that of patients undergoing revision arthroplasty for noninfectious causes.[7] Several patient-specific characteristics have been implicated as risk factors for PJI, and when possible, should be optimized before the index or revision TJA (**Box 1**).[1,2,5,7–11]

PATIENT PRESENTATION

PJI may present as either an acute postoperative infection, an acute hematogenous infection, or as a chronic infection. Patients who develop symptoms within 30 to 90 days postoperatively can be classified as having an acute postoperative infection.[10,12] Those patients with a history of a previously pain-free, well-functioning TJA, and less than 3 to 4 weeks of symptoms, are generally accepted to have an acute infection as a result of hematogenous spread.[12] Often, an infectious origin is not able to be identified in such cases.[13] However, in acute hematogenous infections with a known origin, common sites of origination include the skin and soft tissues, cardiac valves, oral cavity, and urinary tract.[13] Patients who present with new-onset pain or dysfunction after a previously pain-free, functional TJA, and have more than 3 weeks of symptoms, can be diagnosed with chronic PJI.[10]

Common presenting symptoms that should raise suspicion for PJI include persistent wound drainage in the acute postoperative period, joint effusion, fever, acute onset of joint pain after a pain-free interval, chronic postoperative joint pain, persistent stiffness or a decrease in range of motion, and early loosening of the prosthesis.[10,14,15] Occasionally, the initial presentation is that of bacteremia or sepsis, although the workup of these patients is beyond the purview of this article. Patients may also present with a draining sinus tract that communicates with the joint space. In such cases,

---

Box 1
Patient-specific risk factors associated with PJI

- Obesity (BMI > 35)
- Cardiovascular or coronary artery disease
- Peripheral vascular disease
- Diabetes mellitus
- Chronic pulmonary disease
- Renal disease
- Liver disease
- Rheumatologic conditions
- Immunocompromised state
- Psychiatric disorders
- Preoperative anemia
- Perioperative malnutrition
- Tobacco use
- History of avascular necrosis or post-traumatic arthritis
- History of wound infection or PJI

the definitive diagnosis of PJI can be made clinically.[9,10,16] For both patients with a draining sinus tract or who are otherwise suspicious for PJI, further laboratory testing should be initiated promptly. Aside from plain radiographs to rule out alternative diagnoses, imaging modalities are of limited utility in the diagnosis of PJI.[10,14] In 2018, Parvizi and colleagues[16] developed an updated evidence-based, validated algorithm for the diagnosis of PJI (Fig. 1) that can help to guide the preoperative laboratory workup.

PREOPERATIVE WORKUP FOR PERIPROSTHETIC JOINT INFECTION
Erythrocyte Sedimentation Rate and C-Reactive Protein

The serum erythrocyte sedimentation rate (ESR) and high-sensitivity C-reactive protein (CRP) are useful as initial screening tests for PJI, because they exhibit high sensitivity, particularly when interpreted in combination.[9,10,14,16] The optimum cutoff values for an elevated ESR and CRP have been widely debated. Generally, for patients with suspected chronic PJI, ESR values of more than 30 mm/h and CRP values of more than 10 mg/L can be considered a positive screen.[17] The threshold is higher in patients with suspected acute postoperative PJI, because recent surgery is known to cause increases in inflammatory markers. The CRP may remain elevated for up to 6 weeks postoperatively, whereas elevations in the ESR persist for approximately 3 months postoperatively.[18,19] Therefore, in the face of acute PJI, CRP values of greater than

Major criteria (at least one of the following)	Decision
Two positive cultures of the same organism	Infected
Sinus tract with evidence of communication to the joint or visualization of the prosthesis	

		Minor Criteria	Score	Decision
Preoperative Diagnosis	Serum	Elevated CRP _or_ D-Dimer	2	≥6 Infected
		Elevated ESR	1	
	Synovial	Elevated synovial _WBC count or LE_	3	2-5 Possibly Infected [a]
		Positive alpha-defensin	3	
		Elevated synovial PMN (%)	2	0-1 Not Infected
		Elevated synovial CRP	1	

	Inconclusive pre-op score _or_ dry tap [a]	Score	Decision
Intraoperative Diagnosis	Preoperative score	-	≥6 Infected
	Positive histology	3	
	Positive purulence	3	4-5 Inconclusive [b]
	Single positive culture	2	≤3 Not Infected

Fig. 1. New scoring-based definition for PJI. CRP, C-reactive protein; ESR, erythrocyte sedimentation rate; LE, leukocyte esterase; PMN, polymorphonuclear leukocyte; WBC, white blood cell. [a] If inconclusive, operative criteria can be used to fulfill definition for PJI. [b] If inconclusive, consider further molecular diagnostics. (Reprinted from The Journal of Arthroplasty, 33(5), Parvizi J, Tan TL, Goswami K, et al., The 2018 Definition of Periprosthetic Hip and Knee Infection: An Evidence-Based and Validated Criteria, Page 1312, Copyright 2018, with permission from Elsevier.)

100 mg/L should be considered positive.[17] Owing to their low sensitivity, the ESR and CRP values alone are not sufficient for definitive diagnosis of PJI, and elevations should prompt additional testing.[17] In addition to serum ESR and CRP, serum D-dimer has also been shown to be useful in screening for PJI, and is reported to have a higher sensitivity and specificity than ESR and CRP.[20] Given its low cost, the addition of D-dimer when screening with ESR and CRP can lend support in the diagnosis of PJI.

Superficial Swab Cultures

Clinicians unfamiliar with PJI may contemplate the use of swab cultures as another means of screening for PJI in patients with superficial wound drainage or a sinus tract, because they are inexpensive and less invasive tests than synovial fluid testing. However, superficial swab cultures are of limited usefulness in the PJI workup. Only about 50% of superficial swab cultures are consistent with synovial fluid cultures, even when obtained from draining sinus tracts.[21] They have demonstrated higher false-positive and false-negative rates than synovial fluid culture and are more likely to demonstrate multiple organism when positive.[21]

Synovial Fluid Analysis

When serum inflammatory markers are elevated, and suspicion for PJI remains high, arthrocentesis should be performed. When possible, synovial fluid testing should include aerobic and anaerobic cultures, cell count and differential, alpha defensin testing, synovial fluid CRP, and synovial fluid leukocyte esterase (LE).[9,10] Synovial fluid crystal testing can be useful to help rule out crystal arthropathies, which may mimic PJI. In areas with a high prevalence of Lyme disease, consideration should also be given to the addition of synovial fluid Lyme polymerase chain reaction testing, because the traditional synovial fluid culture fails to detect *Borrelia burgdorferi*[22].

On occasion, clinicians may obtain fluid volumes insufficient for completion of all of these testing modalities and will need to prioritize. Synovial fluid LE has demonstrated the greatest specificity, followed by a synovial fluid white blood cell (WBC) count, and therefore may be most useful.[17] Aerobic and anaerobic cultures should also be included, given their propensity to impact treatment in addition to their diagnostic usefulness.

Synovial Fluid Culture

In the medically stable patient, antibiotic administration should be delayed, or held for a minimum of 2 weeks, before synovial fluid culture to decrease the risk of false-negative results.[10] Optimally, synovial fluid specimens should be placed in blood culture medium, which increases yield.[14,23] The clinician should also be cognizant of the potential for infection with atypical pathogens, which are not captured by standard microbial culture, such as fungi, acid-fast bacilli, and low-virulence organisms such as *Propionibacterium acnes*, particularly in immunocompromised patients. Additional microbial testing, including dedicated acid-fast bacilli and fungal cultures, or prolonged incubation of traditional aerobic and anaerobic cultures, may be warranted in such cases. Although the average incubation period for aerobic and anaerobic cultures is 3 to 5 days, incubation for a minimum of 8 days, and as long as 14 days, can increase sensitivity.[23] In addition to prolonged incubation of cultures, multiplex polymerase chain reaction or next-generation sequencing have demonstrated usefulness in identifying low-virulence pathogens often missed with traditional cultures and causative microbes in culture-negative patients.[14,24–26] However, their low sensitivities and high false-positive rates preclude their use as stand-alone diagnostic tests.[24–26]

The microbial profile of periprosthetic infections varies between institutions, by affected joint and with infectious origin.[13,14,23] Gram-positive organisms comprise a majority of culture-positive infections.[14,23] These include *Staphylococcus aureus*, coagulase-negative *Staphylococci*, *Enterococi* and *Streptococi spp.*[13,14,23] Gram-negative organisms have also been implicated in PJI, with *Escherichia coli*, *Pseudomonas spp.*, and *Enterobacter spp.* being the most commonly identifed.[14,23] A significant number of infections, roughly 20%, are polymicrobial, consisting of 2 or more pathogens.[27–29] Around 7% of prosthetic joint infections are culture negative, in which a causative organism is unable to be identified despite meeting the diagnostic criteria for PJI.[14,23,30] Although fungal infections are rare, *Candida albicans* is the pathogen most frequently identified in fungal-associated PJI.[31] *Mycobacterial* prosthetic joint infections are even more rare than fungal infections, but have reported.[29]

Synovial Fluid Cell Counts

In addition to synovial fluid cultures, a cell count with differential, LE and alpha defensin testing can aid in definitive diagnosis of PJI. Of synovial fluid cell counts and differential, synovial fluid WBC count and polymorphonuclear leukocyte percentages are of the greatest value.[25] The optimal thresholds for the diagnosis of PJI have been debated, and vary between acute and chronic infections.[25] For interpretation of the WBC count, a threshold of more than 10,000 cells/μL is commonly used in acute PJI, whereas a cutoff of more than 3,000 cells/μL is accepted for chronic PJI.[25,32] The polymorphonuclear leukocyte percentages threshold in acute infection is around 90%, whereas around 80% is sufficient for chronic PJI.[25,32] Clinicians must use caution when interpreting the automated cell count and differential results in the setting of metal-on-metal prostheses, because results may be falsely elevated secondary to metallosis.[25,33] In such cases, requesting a manual cell count can improve the diagnostic accuracy.[25,33]

Leukocyte Esterase

A relatively new diagnostic test in the setting of PJI, synovial fluid LE is quick and inexpensive. It can easily be performed in the clinic, requiring only centrifugation and analysis using standard urinalysis colorimetric strips.[25,34] It has demonstrated good sensitivity and excellent specificity, outperforming ESR, CRP, and WBC count and differential.[17,25,34] The recommended threshold for a positive LE test is a (++) reading.[25]

Alpha-Defensin

Although also a newer diagnostic test, the synovial fluid biomarker alpha-defensin has become widely available and is increasingly used in diagnosis of PJI. Although it is significantly more costly than the other diagnostic tests, it demonstrated excellent sensitivity and specificity, surpassing other synovial fluid diagnostics, including LE, on both accounts.[25,34] In addition, alpha-defensin testing reacts to a diverse range of pathogens, including gram-positive organisms, gram-negative organisms, atypical bacterial pathogens, fungal pathogens, and polymicrobial infections.[35] However, by virtue of the testing method, alpha-defensin testing cannot be used to discern the specific causative organism.[35]

Two forms of the alpha-defensin test are available, the conventional laboratory enzyme-linked immunosorbent assay testing and a point-of-care lateral flow method.[25,34,36] There are conflicting reports with regard to the efficacy of the enzyme-linked immunosorbent assay method compared with lateral flow. Some studies report a lower performance of the point-of-care lateral flow testing, whereas others report no significant difference in sensitivity and specificity between the 2 testing methods.[25,34,36]

Intraoperative Testing

A prompt preoperative diagnosis of PJI is essential for initiating appropriate and effective treatment. On occasion, definitive diagnosis cannot be achieved preoperatively. In such instances, treatment of presumed PJI should not be delayed. Intraoperative findings may aid in a definitive diagnosis (see **Fig. 1**).[10,14,16] The presence of purulence intraoperatively, as well as positive intraoperative histology using frozen sections, defined as greater than 5 neutrophils per high-powered field in a minimum of 5 high-powered fields, and positive intraoperative cultures, can lend support to or make the diagnosis of PJI.[10,14,16] Two positive intraoperative cultures alone, or 1 positive intraoperative culture consistent with a positive preoperative culture, is sufficient for a definitive diagnosis, regardless of other laboratory findings.[16] Similar to a synovial fluid culture, to increase culture yield, antibiotics should be held for 2 weeks before surgical intervention, particularly when the diagnosis remains equivocal at time of surgery.[10,14,16,23] A minimum of 3, and ideally 5 to 6, intraoperative tissue culture specimens should be obtained.[10,14,16,23] As with a preoperative diagnosis of PJI, intraoperative culture swabs are less reliable for diagnosis.[21,37] In addition to tissue culture, sonication and culture of any explanted components is recommended.[14]

SURGICAL TREATMENT OPTIONS

Because many causative organisms have been known to induce biofilm formation, the cornerstone of treatment for PJI is surgical intervention.[10,14] For patients with acute postoperative or acute hematogenous PJI, debridement, antibiotics, irrigation, and retention of implants (DAIR), with or without an exchange of modular polyethylene components, may be attempted, particularly in the case of less than 1 week of symptoms.[14,38] DAIR may also be attempted outside of these recommendations when patients are at risk for significant morbidity or mortality with more extensive procedures.[14] In some cases, chronic suppressive antibiotics are given as an adjunctive therapy after DAIR, although their impact on long-term outcomes is controversial.[10,14] The success rate of DAIR varies significantly, with reports of rates as high as 90%.[10,39] Worse outcomes have been noted in acute hematogenous infections compared with acute postoperative infections, and in those patients whom are suboptimal candidates but where other procedures are not feasible.[38,40] Notably, failed DAIR negatively impacts outcomes of later staged revision procedures.[38,40]

For patients with either acute or chronic infection, single-stage revision, with resection and reimplantation preformed during a single procedure, may be attempted. although less widely used in the United States, single-stage revision has been shown to have success rates similar to 2-stage revision.[10,14,41] Reinfection rates for a single-stage revision are around 7.8%, whereas rates for a 2-stage revision are around 8.8%.[42] However, a 2-stage revision is still widely considered the gold standard of surgical intervention. It is composed of explanation of the infected prosthesis and placement of antibiotic-impregnated cement spacer, followed by targeted antibiotics, and eventual prosthesis reimplantation.[43]

All surgical procedures should be followed by the administration of targeted antimicrobials. Intravenous agents are used most commonly.[10,14] The optimum duration of therapy ranges from 2 to 6 weeks, depending on the susceptibility of the infecting organism and regional resistance patterns.[10,14] The selection of an appropriate antimicrobial is beyond the scope of this article and is typically done in conjunction with infectious disease specialists.

The risks for failure of revision arthroplasty for infection include, in descending order of importance, previous DAIR, patient history of myocardial infarction, revision index procedure, presence of a sinus tract, culture growth of resistant organism, recent or remote history of smoking, increasing number of prior surgeries other that arthroscopic, elevated preoperative WBC count, elevated body mass index, and an elevated ESR.[43] In rare cases, if infection cannot be eradicated by DAIR, single, or 2-stage revision, amputation or girdlestone may need to be considered[14,44]

SUMMARY

PJI is a rare but devastating complication of total hip and total knee arthroplasty, associated with significant morbidity, and increased 1-year mortality after revision arthroplasty. It may present in the acute postoperative period, or as an acute hematogenous or chronic infection, months to years after index arthroplasty. Several patient-specific risk factors have been identified as contributing to an increased risk of PJI, including modifiable risk factors such as obesity, diabetes mellitus, and smoking. Presenting symptoms of PJI include persistent wound drainage, presence of a sinus tract, joint effusion, fever, acute or chronic joint pain, persistent stiffness, decreased range of motion, or early loosening. A prompt diagnosis of PJI is critical for effective treatment.

The definitive diagnosis can be made clinically if a sinus tract is present. Otherwise, a thorough workup should be undertaken. The initial screening should include serum ESR, CRP, and D-dimer. If the results are elevated or suspicion for PJI remains high, arthrocentesis should be performed to obtain a synovial fluid culture, synovial fluid cell counts with differential, synovial fluid LE, alpha-defensin testing, and synovial fluid ESR. A new diagnostic algorithm using these parameters has been developed to aid in diagnosis. Surgical intervention is the cornerstone of treatment and should not be delayed, even if the diagnosis remains equivocal. An intraoperative finding of purulence, positive intraoperative histology, or positive intraoperative tissue cultures can be used to support the diagnosis of PJI when the preoperative diagnosis is uncertain. Surgical treatment options for PJI include DAIR and a single-stage or 2-stage revision, depending on the chronicity of symptoms. In addition to surgical intervention, targeted antibiotics should be administered for several weeks postoperatively.

ACKNOWLEDGMENTS

The author thanks Dr. Elie Ghanem (Orthopedic Surgeon and Assistant Professor, University of Alabama at Birmingham Health System) for his expertise in both total joint arthroplasty and article preparation, which were influential to this work.

DISCLOSURE

The author has nothing to disclose.

REFERENCES

1. Triantafyllopoulos GK, Soranoglou VG, Memtsoudis SG, et al. Rate and risk factors for periprosthetic joint infection among 36,494 primary total hip arthroplasties. J Arthroplasty 2018;33(4):1166–70.
2. Namba RS, Inacio MCS, Paxton EW. Risk factors associated with deep surgical site infections after primary total knee arthroplasty: an analysis of 56,216 knees. J Bone Joint Surg Am 2013;95(9):775–82.

3. Edwards JR, Peterson KD, Mu Y, et al. National healthcare safety network (NHSN) report: data summary for 2006 through 2008, issued December 2009. Am J Infect Control 2009;37(10):783–805.

4. Kurtz SM, Lau E, Schmier J, et al. Infection burden for hip and knee arthroplasty in the United States. J Arthroplasty 2008;23(7):984–91.

5. Pugely AJ, Martin CT, Gao Y, et al. The incidence of and risk factors for 30-day surgical site infections following primary and revision total joint arthroplasty. J Arthroplasty 2015;30(9):47–50.

6. Boddapati V, Fu MC, Mayman DJ, et al. Revision total knee arthroplasty for periprosthetic joint infection is associated with increased postoperative morbidity and mortality relative to noninfectious revisions. J Arthroplasty 2018;33(2):521–6.

7. Zmistowski B, Karam JA, Durinka JB, et al. Periprosthetic joint infection increases the risk of one-year mortality. J Bone Joint Surg Am 2013;95(24):2177–84.

8. Bozic KJ, Lau E, Kurtz S, et al. Patient-related risk factors for periprosthetic joint infection and postoperative mortality following total hip arthroplasty in Medicare patients. J Bone Joint Surg Am 2012;94(9):794–800.

9. American Academy of Orthopaedic Surgeons. Diagnosis and prevention of periprosthetic joint infections clinical practice guideline. 2019. Available at: https://www.aaos.org/pjiguideline. Accessed May 1, 2020.

10. Osmon DR, Berbari EF, Berendt AR, et al. Diagnosis and management of prosthetic joint infection: clinical practice guidelines by the infectious diseases society of America. Clin Infect Dis 2012;56:1–10.

11. Kunutsor SK, Whitehouse MR, Blom AW, et al, INFORM Team. Patient-related risk factors for periprosthetic joint infection after total joint arthroplasty: a systematic review and meta-analysis. PLoS One 2016;11(3):e0150866.

12. Tsukayama DT, Goldberg VM, Kyle R. Diagnosis and management of infection after total knee arthroplasty. J Bone Joint Surg Am 2003;85:75–80.

13. Rakow A, Perka C, Trampuz A, et al. Origin and characteristics of haematogenous periprosthetic joint infection. Clin Microbiol Infect 2019;25(7):845–50.

14. Tande AJ, Patel R. Prosthetic joint infection. Clin Microbiol Rev 2014;27(2):302-345.

15. Portillo ME, Salvadó M, Alier A, et al. Prosthesis failure within 2 years of implantation is highly predictive of infection. Clin Orthop Relat Res 2013;471(11):3672–8.

16. Parvizi J, Tan TL, Goswami K, et al. The 2018 definition of periprosthetic hip and knee infection: an evidence-based and validated criteria. J Arthroplasty 2018;33(5):1309–14.

17. Shahi A, Tan TL, Kheir MM, et al. Diagnosing periprosthetic joint infection: and the winner is? J Arthroplasty 2017;32(9S):S232-S235.

18. Berbari E, Mabry T, Tsaras G, et al. Inflammatory blood laboratory levels as markers of prosthetic joint infection: a systematic review and meta-analysis. J Bone Joint Surg Am 2010;92(11):2102-2109.

19. Saleh A, George J, Faour M, et al. Serum biomarkers in periprosthetic joint infections. Bone Joint Res 2018;7(1):85–93.

20. Shahi A, Kheir MM, Tarabichi M, et al. Serum D-dimer test is promising for the diagnosis of periprosthetic joint infection and timing of reimplantation. J Bone Joint Surg Am 2017;99(17):1419–27.

21. Tetreault Matthew W, Nathan GW, Vinay KA, et al. Should draining wounds and sinuses associated with hip and knee arthroplasties be cultured? J Arthroplasty 2013;28(8):133–6.

22. Collins KA, Gotoff JR, Ghanem ES. Lyme disease: a potential source for culture-negative prosthetic joint infection. J Am Acad Orthop Surg Glob Res Rev 2017; 1(5):e023.
23. Kheir MM, Tan TL, Ackerman CT, et al. Culturing periprosthetic joint infection: number of samples, growth duration, and organisms. J Arthroplasty 2018; 33(11):3531–6.e1.
24. Morgenstern C, Cabric S, Perka C, et al. Synovial fluid multiplex PCR is superior to culture for detection of low-virulent pathogens causing periprosthetic joint infection. Diagn Microbiol Infect Dis 2018;90(2):115–9.
25. Goswami K, Parvizi J, Maxwell Courtney P. Current recommendations for the diagnosis of acute and chronic PJI for hip and knee-cell counts, alpha-defensin, leukocyte esterase, next-generation sequencing. Curr Rev Musculoskelet Med 2018;11(3):428–38.
26. Tarabichi M, Shohat N, Goswami K, et al. Can next generation sequencing play a role in detecting pathogens in synovial fluid? Bone Joint J 2018;100-B(2):127–33.
27. Tan TL, Kheir MM, Tan DD, et al. Polymicrobial periprosthetic joint infections: outcome of treatment and identification of risk factors. J Bone Joint Surg Am 2016;98(24):2082–8.
28. Aggarwal V, Bakhshi H, Ecker N, et al. Organism profile in periprosthetic joint infection: pathogens differ at two arthroplasty infection referral centers in Europe and in the United States. J Knee Surg 2014;27(05):399–406.
29. Jitmuang A, Yuenyongviwat V, Charoencholvanich K, et al. Rapidly-growing mycobacterial infection: a recognized cause of early-onset prosthetic joint infection. BMC Infect Dis 2017;17(1). https://doi.org/10.1186/s12879-017-2926-3.
30. Tan TL, Kheir MM, Shohat N, et al. Culture-negative periprosthetic joint infection. JB JS Open Access 2018;3(3). https://doi.org/10.2106/jbjs.oa.17.00060.
31. Azzam K, Javad P, Donald J, et al. Microbiological, clinical, and surgical features of fungal prosthetic joint infections: a multi-institutional experience. J Bone Joint Surg Am 2009;91(Suppl 6):142–9.
32. Zahar A, Lausmann C, Cavalheiro C, et al. How reliable is the cell count analysis in the diagnosis of prosthetic joint infection? J Arthroplasty 2018;33(10):3257–62.
33. Yi PH, Cross MB, Moric M, et al. Do serologic and synovial tests help diagnose infection in revision hip arthroplasty with metal-on-metal bearings or corrosion? Clin Orthop Relat Res 2014;473(2):498–505.
34. Chen Y, Kang X, Tao J, et al. Reliability of synovial fluid alpha-defensin and leukocyte esterase in diagnosing periprosthetic joint infection (PJI): a systematic review and meta-analysis. J Orthop Surg Res 2019;14(1). https://doi.org/10.1186/s13018-019-1395-3.
35. Deirmengian C, Kardos K, Kilmartin P, et al. The alpha-defensin test for periprosthetic joint infection responds to a wide spectrum of organisms. Clin Orthop Relat Res 2015;473(7):2229–35.
36. Kuiper JWP, Verberne SJ, Vos SJ, et al. Does the alpha defensin ELISA test perform better than the alpha defensin lateral flow test for PJI Diagnosis? a systematic review and meta-analysis of prospective studies. Clin Orthop Relat Res 2020;478(6):1333–44.
37. Aggarwal VK, Higuera C, Deirmengian G, et al. Swab cultures are not as effective as tissue cultures for diagnosis of periprosthetic joint infection. Clin Orthop Relat Res 2013;471(10):3196–203.
38. Argenson JN, Arndt M, Babis G, et al. Hip and knee section, treatment, debridement and retention of implant: proceedings of international consensus on orthopedic infections. J Arthroplasty 2019;34(2S):S399–419.

39. Ottesen CS, Troelsen A, Sandholdt H, et al. Acceptable success rate in patients with periprosthetic knee joint infection treated with debridement, antibiotics, and implant retention. J Arthroplasty 2019;34(2):365–8.

40. Choo KJ, Austin M, Parvizi J. Irrigation and debridement, modular exchange, and implant retention for acute periprosthetic infection after total knee arthroplasty. JBJS Essent Surg Tech 2019;9(4):e38.1-2.

41. Rowan FE, Donaldson MJ, Pietrzak JR, et al. The role of one-stage exchange for prosthetic joint infection. Curr Rev Musculoskelet Med 2018;11(3):370–9.

42. Kunutsor SK, Whitehouse MR, Lenguerrand E, et al, INFORM Team. Re-infection outcomes following one- and two-stage surgical revision of infected knee prosthesis: a systematic review and meta-analysis. PLoS One 2016;11(3):e0151537.

43. Kheir MM, Tan TL, George J, et al. Development and evaluation of a prognostic calculator for the surgical treatment of periprosthetic joint infection. J Arthroplasty 2018;33(9). https://doi.org/10.1016/j.arth.2018.04.034.

44. Malcolm TL, Gad BV, Elsharkawy KA, et al. Complication, survival, and reoperation rates following girdlestone resection arthroplasty. J Arthroplasty 2015;30(7): 1183–6.

A Comprehensive Overview of Chest Tubes

Holly Zurich, PA-C[a],*, Angela Preda, PA-C[b], Andrew P. Dhanasopon, MD[c]

KEYWORDS

- Chest tube • Tube thoracostomy • Pneumothorax • Pleural effusion • Empyema
- Hemothorax • Air leak • Digital chest drainage

KEY POINTS

- Chest tube thoracostomy is a bedside procedure for the treatment of pleural effusion, empyema, hemothorax, and pneumothorax. Chest tubes also often are placed after routine thoracic and cardiac surgery.
- Different sizes and shapes of chest tubes and types of drainage devices are available, depending on the specific indication.
- Proper chest tube insertion and management are essential to treating the underlying pleural space pathology.

Video content accompanies this article at http://www.physicianassistant.theclinics.com.

INTRODUCTION

The pleural space is defined as the thin, fluid-filled space between the parietal pleura lining the rib cage and the visceral pleura covering the lungs. This pleural space is filled with a thin layer of lubricating serous fluid produced and absorbed by the mesothelium, the epithelial lining of the pleurae. The normal amount of pleural fluid is approximately 0.26 mL/kg of body mass, or approximately 18 mL for a 70-kg adult.[1]

Several pathologies of the pleural space may occur that typically require intervention. Pleural effusions result from infection, inflammation, or malignancy impairing the homeostasis of pleural fluid, leading to its accumulation. This net effect of the accumulation can be a nidus for infection, leading to an empyema, while also causing compressive effects on the lung itself, preventing adequate lung expansion. Hemothorax, or bleeding in the pleural space usually due to trauma, such as rib fractures

[a] Performance Improvement Surgical Services, Yale New Haven Health, 330 Cedar Street, BB205, New Haven, CT 06510, USA; [b] Smilow Cancer Hospital, Yale New Haven Hospital, 330 Cedar Street, BB205, New Haven, CT 06510, USA; [c] Yale University Department of Surgery, Section of Thoracic Surgery, 330 Cedar Street, BB205, New Haven, CT 06510, USA
* Corresponding author.
E-mail address: holly.zurich@ynhh.org

Physician Assist Clin 6 (2021) 239–260
https://doi.org/10.1016/j.cpha.2020.11.008
2405-7991/21/© 2020 Elsevier Inc. All rights reserved.

or penetrating injury, also prevents adequate lung expansion. Similarly, when a bleb on the visceral pleura ruptures, this accumulation of air in the pleural space, or pneumothorax, causes rapid progressive compression of the lung and, if severe enough, leads to hemodynamic consequences, or tension pneumothorax (**Figs. 1–3**).

The net effect of these pathologic processes is the compressive effect on the lung, requiring urgent evacuation of the fluid and/or air to allow lung re-expansion. The resulting pleural-pleural apposition allows for the restoration of lung mechanics. Evacuation success of pleural effusions, empyemas, and hemothoraces depends on the quality of the fluid and presence of loculations, for which instillation of intrapleural fibrinolytics also can be helpful. If air leak persists after pneumothorax evacuation, this signifies bronchopleural or alveolar pleural fistulas[2] for which instillation of sclerosing agents can help pleurodese. Once chest tubes are in place, the drainage amount, character, and presence of air leak are monitored, along with chest radiographs, to determine the degree of success of evacuation and pleural-pleural apposition. Thus, proper technique and management are critical to the success of this treatment. This article reviews common indications, contraindications, chest tube selection and technique, and management, depending on the clinical scenario.

INDICATIONS/CONTRAINDICATIONS

Chest tubes generally are placed by clinicians involved in patient management, such as thoracic and cardiac surgeons, pulmonologists, emergency medicine clinicians, and advanced practice providers. In recent years, image-guided chest tubes also have been part of the routine practice of interventional pulmonologists and interventional radiologists.[3]

Chest tube thoracostomy generally is indicated when the pathologic pleural process causes clinical deterioration and respiratory and/or hemodynamic decompensation. In addition, chest tubes commonly are placed postoperatively in thoracic and cardiac surgery to monitor postoperative fluid, blood, and air from the pleural cavity.

Pleural effusions can result from exudative or transudative disease processes as well as from trauma, as in the case of hemothorax. Parapneumonic pleural effusions

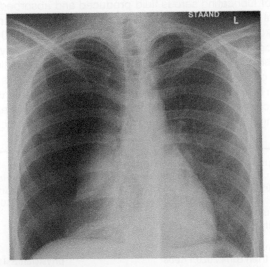

Fig. 1. Pneumothorax.

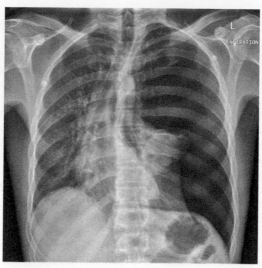

Fig. 2. Tension pneumothorax.

are a type of exudative pleural effusion due to pneumonia and generally are treated with antibiotics and may require chest tube drainage if they do not resolve with the pneumonic process or causes respiratory compromise. Successful evacuation of effusion from the pleural cavity depends on the viscosity of the fluid. More viscous fluid might require the administration of fibrinolytics, such as recombinant tissue plasminogen activator (tPA) and deoxyribonuclease.[1] If the parapneumonic effusion contains debris or loculations, especially when it progresses to empyema, or purulence in the pleural cavity, often surgery is required to clear the process with decortication via minimally invasive (thoracoscopy) or thoracotomy approaches.

Pleural effusions resulting from extrathoracic malignancy often represent stage IV metastatic disease. The goal of treatment of these malignant effusions often is relief

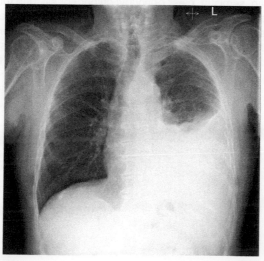

Fig. 3. Pleural effusion.

of respiratory compromise with the maintenance of quality of life. In these circumstances, soft, small indwelling pleural catheters easily can be placed and managed as palliative options.[4]

Another common indication of tube thoracostomy is for pneumothorax causing clinical and respiratory compromise. Pneumothoraces can be categorized as primary (spontaneous), due to ruptured bleb, or secondary due to blunt or penetrating trauma and iatrogenic causes. Iatrogenic pneumothoraces often result from placement of central venous line, transthoracic or transbronchial lung biopsies, or barotrauma suffered during invasive mechanical ventilation.[3] The treatment of pneumothorax depends on the clinical severity and may be observed or more likely require chest tube thoracostomy.[5] If there is persistent air leak after chest tube insertion, patients might require intrapleural sclerosing agents, such as sterile talcum powder, doxycycline, betadine, and so forth, to facilitate pleural-pleural apposition, or surgery via minimally invasive (thoracoscopy) or thoracotomy approach to resect a focal area/bleb causing the air leak with or without concurrent application of a sclerosing agent intraoperatively.[5]

In tension pneumothorax, the air in the pleural cavity exerts sufficient pressure on the great vessels or the heart to cause hemodynamic instability. This situation requires emergent intervention. A life-saving, yet simple, temporizing measure is the insertion of a large-bore needle in the second intercostal space, at the midclavicular line to evacuate the air and decompress the pleural space while chest tube placement is being arranged at bedside.[6]

There are no absolute contraindications to chest tube thoracostomy. Relative contraindications include coagulopathies[7] and the presence of adhesions due to previous chest surgery or pleurodesis and need to be evaluated on a case-by-case basis. Coagulopathies should be corrected prior to chest tube insertion if time allows. If adhesions are encountered during insertion, chest tube placement should be attempted at a different site. Inserting a chest tube over skin abnormalities, such as cellulitis, should be avoided if possible.[2]

CHEST TUBE SELECTION

Chest tubes are long, semistiff, clear polyvinyl chlorideor silicone tubes that are available in various sizes and shapes (**Figs. 4–7**). Chest tube sizes range from 20F to 40F, with common ones 24F to 36F, in straight or angled shapes. Smaller-sized tubes (6F–14F) often are available in a pigtail shape, in which the distal end is coil-shaped. The size and shape of the chest tube used depend on the indication and the patient's body

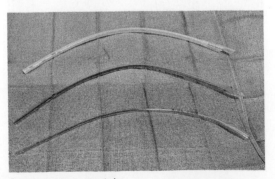

Fig. 4. Chest tube of various sizes, straight.

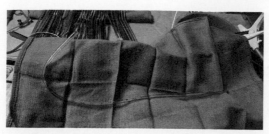

Fig. 5. Angled tube.

habitus but the optimal size of chest tubes used for a specific indication still is a matter of debate and often a function of practitioner preference.[4] The general recommendation is that the larger the volume or viscosity of the fluid to be evacuated, the larger the tube needed. For example, spontaneous pneumothoraces generally are treated using small-bore to medium-bore chest tubes up to 24F. Parapneumonic effusions, hemothoraces, and tubes placed postoperatively in thoracic and cardiac cases typically require large-bore (>24F) chest tubes.

The proximal end of the tube is funnel-shaped to facilitate attachment to tubing that is connected to a drainage device, whereas the distal end is usually tapered and has a series of holes to allow for drainage. A radio-opaque line (blue stripe) runs through the length of the tube with the last proximal hole (sentinel hole), creating a break in the radio-opaque line, which can be visualized on imaging. This safety feature ensures that all holes are inside the chest cavity.

Chest tubes might be positioned differently for specific indications, depending on the medium being drained.[8] Because air tends to rise and collect in the apices, tubes for pneumothoraces usually are directed superiorly toward the apex. Effusions tend to be drawn inferiorly by gravity; thus, posterior and basilar placement with a straight or angled tube is most effective.

CHEST TUBE THORACOSTOMY
Patient History, Examination, Laboratory Tests, and Imaging

Obtaining a good history and reviewing past thoracic surgeries and procedures performed are essential. A patient's medications should be reviewed with attention to anticoagulants and antiplatelet agents. If coagulopathy is suspected, the bleeding risk may be assessed by coagulation studies. The most recent chest imaging (chest

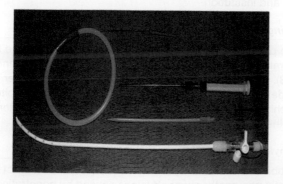

Fig. 6. Pigtail.

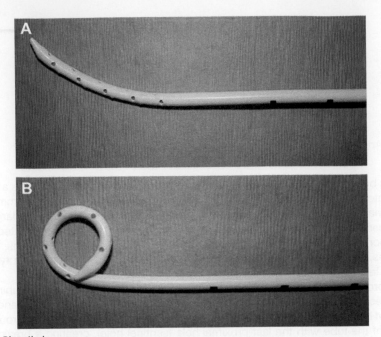

Fig. 7. Pigtail close up.

radiograph or computed tomography) should be reviewed. If recent imaging is not available, at minimum, a chest radiograph should be performed. If a point-of-care ultrasound machine is available, using it to determine and mark the placement site should be considered.

Preparation

After obtaining a written consent, the nurse assigned to the patient should be notified. The equipment/supply pick list in **Box 1** was created as a departmental quality improvement initiative and distributed by the authors' group to various trainees and practitioners at their institution. They have found this list to especially help trainees systematically gather all necessary supplies and equipment beforehand to reduce procedure duration, permit focusing on the procedure itself, and reduce patient (and practitioner) anxiety. The listed chest tube insertion kit has varying contents based on brand and institution.

Patient Positioning

Patients may be positioned supine, with 30° to 45° elevation of the head of the bed with the ipsilateral abducted arm lifted above the head and the hand resting behind the head (**Fig. 8**). A rolled blanket can be placed under the upper back to elevate the ipsilateral side. Patients also may be positioned in lateral decubitus with the clinician standing behind the patient if the tube needs to be directed anteriorly and in front of the patient if the tube is intended to point posteriorly.

Antibiotic Prophylaxis

Prophylactic antibiotics prior to the placement of chest tubes are not necessarily indicated for traumatic pneumothorax or effusions caused by penetrating chest injuries.[9]

Box 1
Equipment and supply pick list for tube thoracostomy

[ ] Chest tube insertion kit

[ ] Antiseptic skin preparation swab

[ ] 20 mL + 10 mL vial 1% lidocaine

[ ] 2 pack sterile towels ×2

[ ] Sterile half-drape

[ ] Chest tube (size dependent on indication)

[ ] Chest drainage system

[ ] Suction setup/tubing

[ ] Sterile gloves/hat/gown

[ ] Sterile water (to fill suction control chamber)

[ ] Tape for pressure dressing

[ ] Tube securement device (optional)

Sedation

Premedication with a short-acting opioid and benzodiazepine should be considered as per floor unit and hospital policies. Care and attention must be paid to dosing based on patient age, weight, and comorbidities.

Anesthesia

The skin, subcutaneous tissues, and parietal pleura at the insertion site as well as the rib periosteum below the insertion site must be anesthetized by local infiltration. Generally, 7 mg/kg of lidocaine with or without epinephrine (1:100,00) is used. In most cases, 20 mL of lidocaine with epinephrine can be prepared, with an additional 10 mL available if needed.

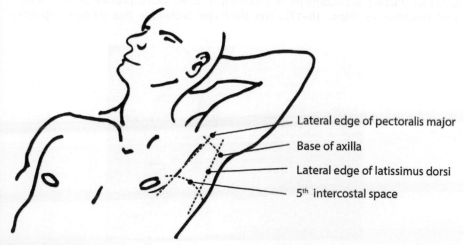

Lateral edge of pectoralis major

Base of axilla

Lateral edge of latissimus dorsi

5th intercostal space

Fig. 8. Patient positioning/safe triangle.

Insertion Site

When inserting a chest tube, the intended final position of the tube determines where to make the incision. Chest tubes commonly are inserted on the ipsilateral chest wall between the anterior and midaxillary line at the fourth or fifth intercostal space within the safe triangle formed by the lateral border of the pectoralis major muscle, the lateral border of the latissimus dorsi muscles, the fifth intercostal space, and the base of the axilla. A less common insertion site is the second or third intercostal space at the mid-clavicular line; however, this site is less well tolerated. Tubes inserted posterior to the latissimus muscle also are not well tolerated. If the intended insertion site is close to a site where adhesions are anticipated, an alternative approach must be planned.

Techniques

Blunt dissection

Blunt dissection is the most widely used technique for tube thoracostomy (**Figs. 9–14**). An incision wide enough to accommodate the index finger (2–3 cm) is made parallel to and over the rib or the intercostal space inferior to the pleural entry site. Avoiding the inferior edge of the rib, blunt dissection of the subcutaneous tissue and intercostal muscles is achieved using a clamp (eg, curved Kelly clamp). By creating a track that is angled superiorly, the pleural space is entered directly above the superior edge of the rib, using the tip of the clamp. Creating this tract both angles the chest tube superiorly to reach the apex and provides a better seal against an air leak, because the tube has to traverse a longer distance in the chest wall. Digital exploration of the pleural space is performed using the index finger to sweep for adherence of the lung to the pleura, because this impedes the passage of the tube and could lead to extrathoracic placement or visceral injury. The clamp then is used to guide the distal end of the tube into the pleural cavity to achieve a basilar or apical position for effusion or air drainage, respectively. One to 2 sutures can be placed to anchor the tube in place and to assist in closing the incision around the tube. Occlusive dressing is prepared by wrapping the tube with Vaseline-impregnated gauze and cover sponge that might be reinforced with tape.

Seldinger technique

Although blunt dissection has been the mainstay of chest tube placement, the Seldinger technique has become more prevalent in recent years, popularized by nonsurgical practitioners (**Figs. 15–17**). The Seldinger technique has gained popularity

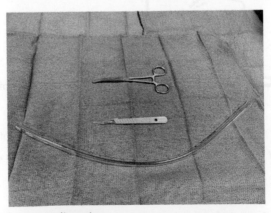

Fig. 9. Instruments for blunt dissection.

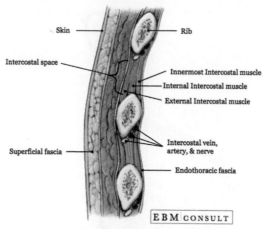

Fig. 10. Blunt dissection illustration. "Image Provided by EBM Consult".

because it causes less damage to the tissue, leading to improved pain level and a less visible scar.[10] The Seldinger technique uses a guide wire that is threaded into the pleural space. After a series of dilators are passed into the thoracic cavity, the chest tube is inserted over the guide wire. Although better tolerated than the blunt dissection, the Seldinger technique does not allow for the digital manipulation of the pleural space and affords limited ability to guide the tube. The Seldinger technique requires certainty that the intended insertion space is large enough, confirmed by imaging (ultrasound or computed tomography) or the aspiration of fluid from the pleural space.

Postprocedure Assessment

The chest tube connection to the tubing of the drainage device should be secured by tape or zip ties and the drainage device should be inspected for tidaling, signifying patency and correct placement position within the pleural space (**Fig. 18**). Vital signs,

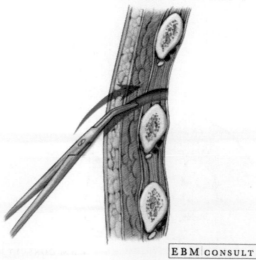

Fig. 11. Blunt dissection illustration. "Image Provided by EBM Consult".

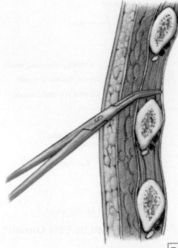

EBM CONSULT

Fig. 12. Blunt dissection illustration. "Image Provided by EBM Consult".

including pulse oximetry, should be assessed postprocedure as well as lung sounds, by auscultating bilaterally. A stat chest radiograph must be obtained to confirm the placement and functioning via the resolution of pneumothorax and evacuation of the effusion. **Table 1** is a checklist created as part of departmental quality improvement initiative, discussed previously, to ensure that trainees and practitioners utilize standardized steps to reduce variation and errors.

DRAINAGE DEVICES
Three-Chamber Drainage Devices

The modern 3-chamber drainage device was modeled after the traditional water seal drainage systems that consisted of 3 bottles connected in line and consisted of a

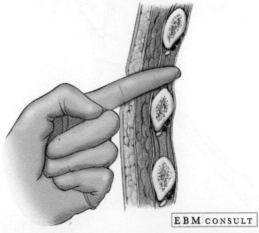

EBM CONSULT

Fig. 13. Blunt dissection illustration. "Image Provided by EBM Consult".

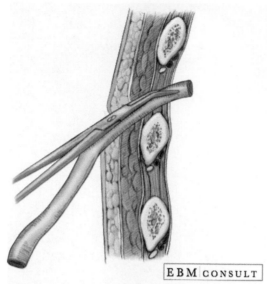

Fig. 14. Blunt dissection illustration. "Image Provided by EBM Consult".

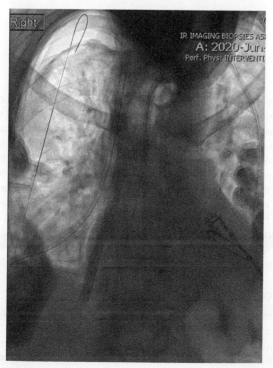

Fig. 15. Seldinger technique.

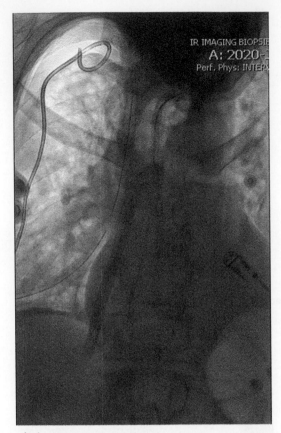

Fig. 16. Seldinger technique.

collection chamber, a water-seal chamber, and a suction control chamber (**Fig. 19**). After the pleural fluid is collected in the collection chamber, the next water seal chamber works as a 1-way valve by having the tubing immersed in a few centimeters of water, so that air can exit by bubbling through the water but atmospheric air cannot pass into the chest. Positive pressure in the pleural space generates bubbles that can be observed in the water seal chamber, which defines an air leak. The air leak is best observed when the patient coughs or performs a Valsalva maneuver, because these actions generally release the air trapped in the pleural cavity. Three-chamber chest drainage devices have 3 modes: suction, water-seal, and clamping (discussed later). The suction is controlled by filling the suction control chamber to 20 cm H_2O and is independent of the degree of wall suction applied. Suction also is influenced by the level of fluid in the tubing and the position of the device relative to the patient.[11]

Digital Drainage Devices

Digital portable drainage devices have been available since 2007, but more widespread use came in 2014, with the introduction of Thopaz+ (Medela, McHenry, Illinois), which provides quantitative measurement of the air leak and fluid drained over time (**Fig. 20**).[12] These data are provided by the device via a display every minute and can be trended for 24 hours. Another advantage of digital systems is the ability to

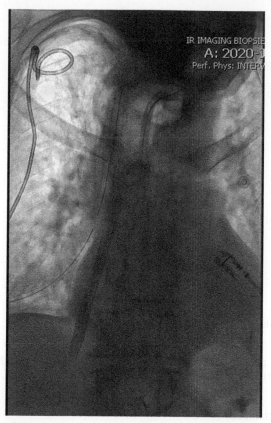

Fig. 17. Seldinger technique.

maintain a strict range of pleural pressure within a preset value.[13] Studies have found that post–lung resection, patients managed with a digital system experienced a shorter duration of chest tube placement, had shorter hospital stays,[4,14] and were more satisfied with their experience compared with patients who were assigned to traditional drainage devices.[15] Relative to traditional drainage systems, however, there is a greater capital investment needed with the digital devices and maintenance and greater cost of the disposable components (drainage box and tubing), and they may be more prone to clogging with debris with less ability to strip the tubing due to the stiffer material. At the authors' institution, the use of either traditional or digital drainage systems has been strategized based on the indication. For example, for drainage of pleural space infections and hemothoraces and postoperative cardiac surgery, a traditional drainage system tends to be used, which is effective at the evacuation of debris, blood, and their clearance from the tubing. For pneumothoraces or straightforward lung resections, the digital drainage system can be used, particularly to monitor the trend in the quantitative air leak over time.

Portable Traditional Drainage Devices (Atrium Express Mini 500, Pneumostat, and Heimlich Valve)

For patients who are discharged from the hospital with a chest tube, there are a variety of portable drainage systems that can be used, depending on the anticipated volume

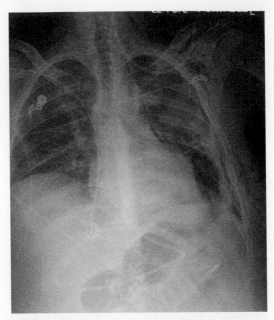

Fig. 18. Angled tube in left chest.

of fluid drainage per day and the comfort level of the patient and practitioner with maintenance and monitoring (Atrium mini [**Fig. 21**]; pneumostat [**Fig. 22**]; and Heimlich valve [**Fig. 23**]).

Atrium Express Mini 500

The Atrium Express Mini 500 (Getinge, Gothenburg, Sweden) is a portable dry seal system that can store up to 500 mLs of fluid[16]; thus, it is useful in situations when

Table 1
Checklist for chest tube thoracostomy

Procedural Checklists		
Preprocedure	**Procedure**	**Postprocedure**
[ ] Review labs (PT/PTT, Plt)	[ ] Time out	[ ] Stitch tube
[ ] Review prior chest surgery	[ ] Medications	[ ] Dressing
[ ] Review meds (anticoagulants, antiplatelet agents)	(consider IV opioids, IV benzodiazepines	[ ] Secure tube connection to drainage device (tape or zip tie)
[ ] Review imaging	as per floor policy	[ ] Chest drainage system to
[ ] Consent	if ICU/ED setting)	suction
[ ] Consider US- mark site	[ ] Position patient	[ ] Assess ± air leak/quality and
[ ] Notify RN/primary team	[ ] Mark site	quantity of drainage
	[ ] Universal protocol/ sterile technique	[ ] Stat CXR—review to confirm proper placement
		[ ] Procedural note
		[ ] Place appropriate orders (chest tube care, daily CXR)
		[ ] Assess glove, dispose of sharps

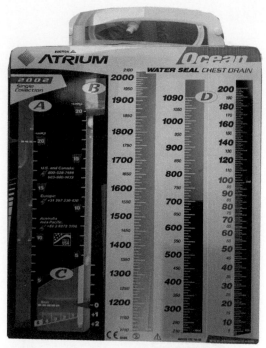

Fig. 19. Atrium with labels.

air and fluid drainage both are anticipated, such as post–thoracic surgery. This is approximately a quarter of the size and volume capacity of the full-size Atrium drainage systems, making it more convenient for home use or patient mobilization.

Pneumostat

The Pneumostat Chest Drain Valve (Getinge, Gothenburg, Sweden) is a smaller, single-use dry seal chest drain valve with the capacity to hold a small amount of drained fluid (30 mL) that allows for easy mobility of patients treated for pneumothorax.[17]

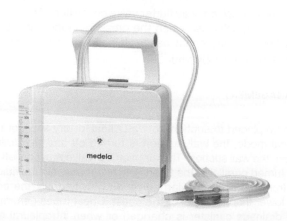

Fig. 20. Medelas.

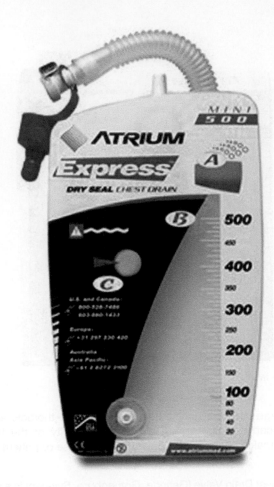

Fig. 21. Atrium mini.

Heimlich valve

The Heimlich valve is a passive 1-way flutter valve consisting of a soft rubber tube that allows air to escape but collapses when the pressure in the chest cavity drops and thus prevents airflow into the chest cavity. If needed, the Heimlich valve can be attached to suction or a drainage bag.[18]

CHEST TUBE MANAGEMENT
Modes

Chest tubes can be placed to suction, to water seal (or dry seal), or be clamped. To use the water seal mode, the wall suction is turned off and the drainage system is disconnected from the wall suction. The air overflow valve must be left in the open position (stopcock turned parallel to the tubing). In this mode, air and fluid are allowed to passively drain from the chest, relying solely on gravity; thus, the collection device must be placed lower than the level of the chest. Chest tubes generally are clamped when the chest drainage canister is changed or when intrapleural medications are instilled. Chest tubes also may be clamped prior to removal. Clamping the chest

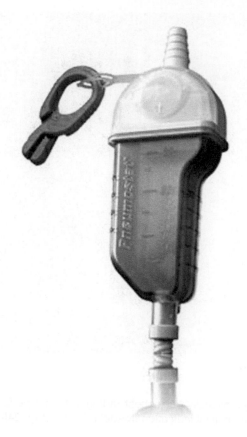

Fig. 22. Pneumostat

tube leads to a pleural space with no outlet for the evacuation of fluid or air; thus, the patient must be monitored closely for clinical changes, and, generally, a chest film is obtained within 1 hour to 3 hours of clamping. In the Medela Thopaz$^+$ chest drainage system, suction is generated by the stand-alone device. Instead of a water seal, Thopaz$^+$ devices have a physio mode, in which suction is turned off and no negative pressure is generated above what is physiologic.

Observation

Chest tube drainage systems generally are monitored for the presence of an air leak and the quality and quantity of fluid in the collection chamber by both nursing and covering providers. To assess for an air leak in the 3-chamber system, the provider can observe bubbling in the water seal chamber. This chamber is marked 1 to 5 (right to left, with 5 being the highest) to allow for easier quantification of the air leak (Videos 1 and 2).

Other things to look for are kinked chest tubes, whether the dressing is intact and dry, and whether the chest tube is secured to the chest wall. Patients also frequently are assessed for subcutaneous emphysema, by palpating the skin surrounding the insertion site. On the Medela Thopaz device, the air leak is quantified and can be followed over time, observing the graph displayed. Throughout the course of monitoring

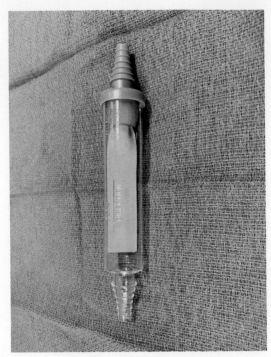

Fig. 23. Heimlich valve.

chest tube drainage, typically daily chest radiographs are performed to evaluate for the resolution of the original indication (Medela display [**Fig. 24**]).

Deciding When to Remove

The timing of chest tube removal depends on the original indication for placement and the institution-specific and practitioner-specific thresholds and criteria met. For example, for parapneumonic effusions, once the daily amount has subsided, the lung has re-expanded, and clinical indicators infection has resolved, the chest tube is removed. In cases of pneumothorax, the chest tube generally is placed on suction for 24 hours or until the air leak resolves. Some clinicians place the tube on water seal and/or clamp and reassess before removal. A survey of 409 pulmonologists and thoracic surgeons showed that the clinicians' preference was divided equally between either removing the chest tube after performing a clamping trial for 24 hours or removing the chest tube without a clamping trial immediately after air leak cessation.[19] There appears to be no significant difference in clinical outcomes. Communication with the patient's surgeon is critical to determine the optimal timing of tube removal.

Removal

During a normal breath cycle, the pleural space is at a negative pressure relative to atmospheric pressure, with the most negative interpleural pressure at end inspiration. Chest tubes generally are removed during exhalation or at end exhalation because of the reduced pressure gradient during these periods. This avoids the incision site sucking in air leading to the re-expansion of the pneumothorax. In patients whose mental status does not allow for slow exhalation, humming could be substituted. Some

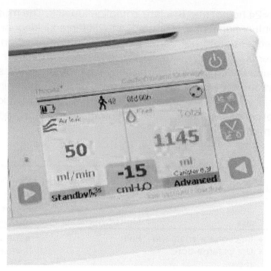

Fig. 24. Medela display.

clinicians remove tubes at end-inspiration but a small prospective study of 102 pa-tients found no difference in the rate of postremoval pneumothorax between the end-inspiration and end-expiration removal groups.[20] After the removal of anchoring sutures, the entry site is covered by an occlusive dressing. This dressing should remain in place for 48 hours. For smaller tubes placed by the Seldinger technique, min-imal coverage might suffice. A post-pull radiograph may be obtained in 2 hours to 4 hours to assess for the presence of recurrent pneumothorax.

MANAGEMENT OF CHEST TUBES AFTER LUNG RESECTION

Whether to place the chest tube to suction versus water seal in a postoperative patient is institution-specific and surgeon-specific and dependent on the conduct of the oper-ation. Two of 3 meta-analyses favor the application of suction versus water seal. In 1 meta-analysis of 8 trials of 1139 patients, investigators showed no difference in the incidence of prolonged air leak, although there was significant heterogeneity of the tri-als.[21] Another meta-analysis of 7 trials found no differences in terms of incidence of prolonged air leak, duration of chest tube placement, or hospital stay when chest tubes were placed to suction or water seal, although suction appeared to significantly reduce the incidence of pneumothorax compared with water seal.[22] A meta-analysis of 10 randomized controlled trials of 1601 post–pulmonary surgery patients found that the addition of external suction compared with water seal reduced the occurrence of postoperative pneumothorax and other cardiopulmonary complications while increasing the duration of chest drainage but had no effect on air leak duration, the occurrence of prolonged air leak, or the length of hospitalization.[23] Chest tubes that were inserted for the indication of postoperative fluid and air drainage generally are removed, with the cessation of air leak and decreasing amounts of fluid that is less than 200 mL to 400 mL in a 24-hour period if no abnormalities are noted on imaging.

COMPLICATIONS

According to a prospective study that included 106 patients with various indications, tube thoracostomy performed by trained personnel carries a 3% early complication risk (presenting in <24 hours) and 8% late complication risk. The most common complications were nonfunctional chest tubes due to clotting, kinking, or dislodgement.[24] Although the investigators did not consider pain as a complication, it is a common complaint by patients. Although rare, injury to visceral organs or great vessels is one of the most serious complications and may warrant emergent surgical intervention. Ectopic insertion may injure any intrathoracic or intra-abdominal organ but the most commonly injured structures are the lung, heart, diaphragm, and great vessels.[25] **Table 2** lists complications, causes, signs/symptoms to monitor, and ways to prevent or intervene to correct.

Table 2
Complications of chest tube thoracostomy

Complication	Cause	Signs/Symptoms	Prevention/ Intervention
Pain with insertion	• Inadequate analgesia • Use of large-bore tube • Posteriorly located tube	Pain	• Titrate sedation/ analgesia. • Use smaller tube. • Avoid inferior edge of rib.
Intercostal neuralgia	Trauma to the neurovascular bundle	Persistent pain	• Avoid inferior edge of rib.
Increasing pneumothorax (while the tube still is intrathoracic)	• Accumulation of air without the ability to escape • Kinking • Clogging	• Acute chest pain • Dyspnea • Tachypnea	• Monitor for patency. • Flush with saline, tPA ± DNase.
Recurrent pneumothorax (after tube removal)	• Premature removal/ clamping • Air entry through chest tube site	• Acute chest pain • Dyspnea • Tachypnea	• Application of occlusive dressing • Remove during/at end exhalation. • Insert new chest tube if clinically significant.
Dislodged tube	• Inadequate securement • Accidental tension	• The tube has slipped out or detached from the drainage system.	• Avoid diagonal wrapping of the tube with suture when securing. • Application of sterile occlusive dressing taped down on 3 sides.
Re-expansion pulmonary edema	>1–1.5 L fluid drainage in <30 min	• Dyspnea • Cough • Decreased O_2 sat • Chest radiograph finding	• Remove <1L fluid in 30 min. • Supplemental O_2
Local infection	Emergent insertion	Redness, purulent discharge and pain at the insertion site	+/− Antibiotics
Ectopic position	Perforation of the lung, heart, great vessels, diaphragm or other visceral organs	Pain, +/− hemodynamic instability, depending on the organ	• Digital exploration to sweep pleura • Image guidance

DISCUSSION AND SUMMARY

Although there are many variations in practice, the critical concepts required for a successful outcome include recognition of the pleural space pathology for which a tube thoracostomy is helpful, mobilizing resources based on urgency, selection of the proper tube and drainage device, safe and effective insertion technique, appropriate tube management, and prevention and recognition of complications. The same principles apply to patients who have undergone routine thoracic and cardiac surgery, with an emphasis on postoperative management and monitoring for complications. The patient who has had a successful treatment with chest tube thoracostomy should have immediate near-resolution of underlying pleural space pathology, recovery of respiratory mechanics, and tolerable pain that continues to subside. If none of these conditions is met, it behooves the practitioner to investigate for potential complications or consider if more invasive surgical intervention is necessary to correct the pathology. Institutional policies, personal preferences, and even dogma may dictate some of the details of management, such as tube size, insertion location and technique, periprocedural analgesics and/or anxiolytics, daily monitoring, and criteria for tube removal and follow-up. Regardless of details, adherence to sound technical principles and appropriate management lead to a good patient-centered outcome.

DISCLOSURE

The authors have nothing to disclose.

REFERENCES

1. Ferreiro L, Porcel JM, Bielsa S, et al. Management of pleural infections. Expert Rev Respir Med 2018;12(6):521–35.
2. Venuta F, Diso D, Anile M, et al. Chest tubes: generalities. Thorac Surg Clin 2017; 27(1):1–5.
3. Loiselle A, Parish JM, Wilkens JA, et al. Managing iatrogenic pneumothorax and chest tubes. J Hosp Med 2013;8(7):402–8.
4. Porcel JM. Chest tube drainage of the pleural space: a concise review for pulmonologists. Tuberc Respir Dis (Seoul) 2018;81(2):106–15.
5. Terzi E, Zarogoulidis K, Kougioumtzi I, et al. Acute respiratory distress syndrome and pneumothorax. J Thorac Dis 2014;6(Suppl 4):S435–42.
6. Drinhaus H, Annecke T, Hinkelbein J. Chest decompression in emergency medicine and intensive care. Anaesthesist 2016;65(10):768–75.
7. Gilbert TB, McGrath BJ, Soberman M. Chest tubes: indications, placement, management, and complications. J Intensive Care Med 1993;8(2):73–86.
8. Mahmood K, Wahidi MM. Straightening out chest tubes. Clin Chest Med 2013; 34(1):63–71.
9. Bosman A, de Jong MB, Debeij J, et al. Systematic review and meta-analysis of antibiotic prophylaxis to prevent infections from chest drains in blunt and penetrating thoracic injuries. Br J Surg 2012;99(4):506–13.
10. McElnay PJ, Lim E. Modern techniques to insert chest drains. Thorac Surg Clin 2017;27(1):29–34.
11. Refai M, Brunelli A, Varela G, et al. The values of intrapleural pressure before the removal of chest tube in non-complicated pulmonary lobectomies. Eur J Cardiothorac Surg 2012;41(4):831–3.
12. 10 Years of Digital Chest Drainage. The J mHealth2018.

13. Inc. M. Thopaz digital chest drainage and monitoring system. Available at: https://www.medelahealthcare.ca/solutions/cardiothoracic-drainage/thopaz. Accessed May 19, 2020.

14. Miller DL, Helms GA, Mayfield WR. Digital drainage system reduces hospitalization after video-assisted thoracoscopic surgery lung resection. Ann Thorac Surg 2016;102(3):955–61.

15. Pompili C, Detterbeck F, Papagiannopoulos K, et al. Multicenter international randomized comparison of objective and subjective outcomes between electronic and traditional chest drainage systems. Ann Thorac Surg 2014;98(2):490–6 [discussion 496–97].

16. Atrium Getinge. Express Mini 500. 2020. Available at: https://www.getinge.com/us/product-catalog/express-mini-500-mobile-dry-seal-drain/. Accessed May 17, 2020.

17. Chan KY, Fikri-Abdullah M, Sajjad M, et al. Outpatient treatment of spontaneous pneumothorax using an improved pocket sized Heimlich valve. Med J Malaysia 2003;58(4):597–9.

18. Gogakos A, Barbetakis N, Lazaridis G, et al. Heimlich valve and pneumothorax. Ann Transl Med 2015;3(4):54.

19. Baumann MH, Strange C. The clinician's perspective on pneumothorax management. Chest 1997;112(3):822–8.

20. Bell RL, Ovadia P, Abdullah F, et al. Chest tube removal: end-inspiration or end-expiration? J Trauma 2001;50(4):674–7.

21. Lang P, Manickavasagar M, Burdett C, et al. Suction on chest drains following lung resection: evidence and practice are not aligned. Eur J Cardiothorac Surg 2016;49(2):611–6.

22. Coughlin SM, Emmerton-Coughlin HM, Malthaner R. Management of chest tubes after pulmonary resection: a systematic review and meta-analysis. Can J Surg 2012;55(4):264–70.

23. Zhou J, Chen N, Hai Y, et al. External suction versus simple water-seal on chest drainage following pulmonary surgery: an updated meta-analysis. Interact Cardiovasc Thorac Surg 2019;28(1):29–36.

24. Collop NA, Kim S, Sahn SA. Analysis of tube thoracostomy performed by pulmonologists at a teaching hospital. Chest 1997;112(3):709–13.

25. Filosso PL, Guerrera F, Sandri A, et al. Errors and complications in chest tube placement. Thorac Surg Clin 2017;27(1):57–67.

Chest Tube Drainage in the Age of COVID-19

Andrew P. Dhanasopon, MD[a], Holly Zurich, PA-C[b],*, Angela Preda, PA-C[c]

KEYWORDS

- COVID-19 • SARS-CoV-2 • Chest tube • Tube thoracostomy • Pneumothorax
- Barotrauma • Pleural effusion

KEY POINTS

- Chest tubes are commonly placed at the bedside for the treatment of pneumothorax and/or pleural effusion for the COVID-19 patient.
- Barotrauma caused by mechanical ventilation can manifest as a pneumothorax, which is commonly treated with tube thoracostomy.
- Pleural air released by tube thoracostomy is a potential source of airborne infection owing to aerosolization of the severe acute respiratory syndrome coronavirus 2 virus.
- Various strategies are emerging to reduce the risk of infection associated with exposure to pleural air.

INTRODUCTION

Chest tube thoracostomy in patients with airborne precautions requires special consideration, as air leaks are a potential source of airborne infection. Although no definitive guidance exists regarding the potential aerosolization of the severe acute respiratory syndrome coronavirus 2 (SARS-CoV-2),[1] chest tube insertion, management, and removal are all potentially aerosol-generating procedures and may create a risk of exposure for health care personnel.

COVID-19 is a respiratory syndrome whose clinical manifestations range from asymptomatic to severe interstitial pneumonia and acute respiratory distress syndrome (ARDS).[2] A metaanalysis of 19 observational studies showed that about one-third of hospitalized COVID-19 patients develop ARDS (32.8% [95% confidence interval 13.7–51.8]).[3] Pneumothorax appears to be a frequent complication of ARDS in general, with 1 study demonstrating the incidence to be 48.8%.[4] The proportion of mechanically ventilated COVID-19 patients with ARDS who suffer pneumothorax

[a] Department of Surgery, Section of Thoracic Surgery, Yale University, 330 Cedar Street, BB205, New Haven, CT 06520, USA; [b] Performance Improvement Surgical Services, Yale New Haven Health, 330 Cedar Street, BB205, New Haven, CT 06520, USA; [c] Smilow Cancer Hospital, Yale New Haven Hospital, 330 Cedar Street, BB205, New Haven, CT 06520, USA
* Corresponding author.
E-mail address: holly.zurich@ynhh.org

Physician Assist Clin 6 (2021) 261–265
https://doi.org/10.1016/j.cpha.2020.11.011
2405-7991/21/© 2020 Elsevier Inc. All rights reserved.

physicianassistant.theclinics.com

because of barotrauma is anticipated to be similar, but is not yet known.[4,5] The development of pneumothorax in ARDS has been associated with as much as 20% higher mortality compared with those without pneumothorax.[6] Thus, prompt recognition and treatment of pneumothorax in any mechanically ventilated patient, and particularly in patients with ARDS and COVID-19-related ARDS, can prevent further respiratory and hemodynamic deterioration.

The following risk mitigation strategies have been proposed and are under review at the authors' institution to minimize exposure to pleural air during chest tube placement in the COVID-19 patient. These modifications of the standard insertion technique were developed in parallel and in correspondence with members of the American Association for the Surgery of Trauma (AAST) Acute Care Surgery and Critical Care Committee. Please refer to their guidelines for further details.[7]

CHEST TUBE INSERTION IN THE COVID-19 PATIENT
Triaging

- Elective insertion should be postponed until COVID-19 testing can be performed if possible.
- In patients with unknown COVID-19 status when chest tube placement is required on an urgent or emergent basis or in a patient with confirmed COVID-19-positive status, the procedure should be performed in a negative-pressure airborne precaution isolation room.

Preparation

- Use appropriate personal protective equipment for aerosol-generating procedures.
- Bring only essential equipment into the room.
- Leave backup equipment outside of the room with an assistant positioned outside.
- Set up equipment outside of the room as much as possible, including the chest tube drainage system.
- The procedure should be performed by an experienced practitioner, with minimal nonessential personnel present. The AAST guidelines recommend establishment of a dedicated thoracic procedure team.[7]

Mechanically Ventilated Patients

- If the patient is mechanically ventilated, consider the use of neuromuscular blockade to prevent coughing and to facilitate holding respirations while entering the pleural space and until placement of tube. Both coughing and respirations could expel potentially infectious pleural air.

Insertion

- Fully drape the entire patient instead of the half drape commonly used for this procedure.
- When possible, use a small-diameter pigtail catheter (eg, 14F) with percutaneous Seldinger technique. If a large-bore tube is required, use a smaller incision and a tunneled approach to reduce the amount of potentially infectious air leak.
- Clamp the tube before insertion to prevent pleural air escaping via the newly inserted chest tube.
- Attach the tube to the previously prepared chest tube management system tubing for egress of air from the thoracic cavity.
- Close the skin incision around the tube to prevent air leakage around the tube.

Prone-Positioned Patients

- Prone positioning is used to improve lung mechanics and gas exchange by enhancing lung recruitment.[8] This technique is used as an adjunct in the management of ARDS patients, including mechanically ventilated COVID-19 patients.
- When prone-positioned patients require chest tube thoracostomy, place a rolled blanket to elevate the lateral chest and insert the chest tube as close to the mid-axillary line as possible within the "safe triangle" (**Fig. 1**) to avoid kinking of the tube.

CHEST DRAINAGE SYSTEM MANAGEMENT IN THE COVID-19 PATIENT

When possible, the drainage system should be placed on suction. In this setup, the suction canister and medical gas vacuum lines exhaust in a manner similar to a negative pressure room. When the system is placed on water seal and disconnected from wall suction, air leaking from the lung can flow into the drainage system and into the room. Thus, the use of a water seal should be avoided. Patients, however, might need to be transported for various reasons, and maintaining wall suction might not be feasible. Although neither 3-chamber nor digital chest drainage systems are equipped with viral filters, the 3-chamber system can be easily modified using the following options to offer potential viral protection to make water seal safe.

In-Line Viral Filters

Repurposed ventilator or smoke-evacuation viral in-line filters may be attached in between the 3-chamber device and the wall canister. Filters that have been proposed by other groups include the in-line BILF-150/200 filter (Buffalo Filter LLC) originally used in surgical smoke evacuation[7] or a ventilator filter, such as the Air-Life 303EU bacterial/viral filter (Carefusion)[9] or Filta-Guard (Intersurgical Ltd)[1] (**Figs. 2** and **3**).

- Consider adding dilute bleach in the water seal chamber with or without the filter in the 3-chamber chest drainage system.

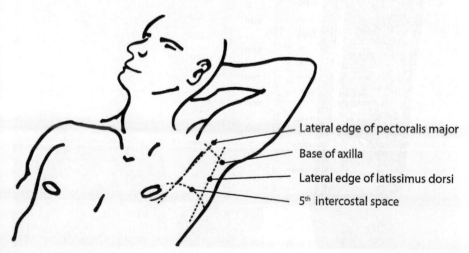

Lateral edge of pectoralis major

Base of axilla

Lateral edge of latissimus dorsi

5th intercostal space

Fig. 1. Safe triangle.

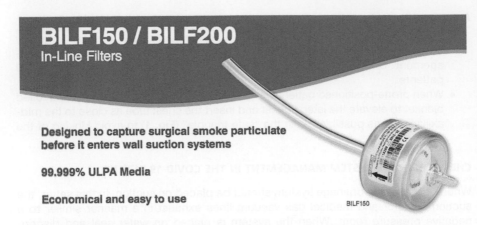

Designed to capture surgical smoke particulate before it enters wall suction systems

99.999% ULPA Media

Economical and easy to use

BILF150

Fig. 2. BILF150/BILF200 filter.

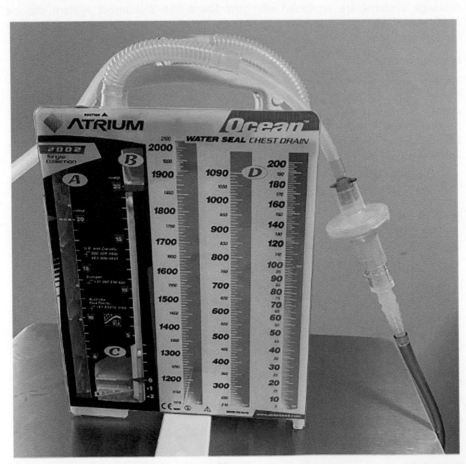

Fig. 3. Atrium Ocean with bacterial/viral filter.

CHEST TUBE REMOVAL

- Minimize staff in the room and use personal protective equipment appropriate for an aerosol-generating procedure.
- Place an occlusive dressing over the tube site, reinforced by pressure dressing.
- Carefully dispose of the chest tube and the drainage device and doubling the biohazard bag.

SUMMARY

Chest tube thoracostomy for patients with COVID-19 warrant special consideration given the mode of transmission of the SARS-CoV-2 virus and the aerosolizing nature of the procedure itself. Proper preparation, personal protective equipment, modified techniques, and drainage maintenance are critical to minimizing exposure to health care personnel.

DISCLOSURE

The authors have nothing to disclose.

REFERENCES

1. Bilkhu R VA, Saftic I, Billè A. COVID-19: chest drains with air leak – the silent 'super spreader'? April 2020.
2. Wang D, Hu B, Hu C, et al. Clinical characteristics of 138 hospitalized patients with 2019 novel coronavirus–infected pneumonia in Wuhan, China. JAMA 2020; 323(11):1061–9.
3. Rodriguez-Morales AJ, Cardona-Ospina JA, Gutiérrez-Ocampo E, et al. Clinical, laboratory and imaging features of COVID-19: a systematic review and meta-analysis. Trav Med Infect Dis 2020;34:101623.
4. Aiolfi A, Biraghi T, Montisci A, et al. Management of persistent pneumothorax with thoracoscopy and blebs resection in COVID-19 patients. Ann Thorac Surg 2020; 110(5):e413–5.
5. Ioannidis G, Lazaridis G, Baka S, et al. Barotrauma and pneumothorax. J Thorac Dis 2015;(suppl 1):S38–43.
6. Gattinoni L, Bombino M, Pelosi P, et al. Lung structure and function in different stages of severe adult respiratory distress syndrome. JAMA 1994;271(22):1772–9.
7. Pieracci FM, Burlew CC, Spain D, et al. Tube thoracostomy during the COVID-19 pandemic: guidance and recommendations from the AAST acute care surgery and critical care committees. Trauma Surg Acute Care Open 2020;5(1):e000498..
8. Fan E, Del Sorbo L, Goligher EC, et al. An official American Thoracic Society/European Society of Intensive Care Medicine/Society of Critical Care Medicine Clinical Practice Guideline: mechanical ventilation in adult patients with acute respiratory distress syndrome. Am J Respir Crit Care Med 2017;195(9):1253–63.
9. Stephan Soder SK. Creating a COVID-19 safe chest tube drainage system. 2020. Available at: https://www.sts.org/sites/default/files/Chest tube drainage system for CoVid-19 (1) (1).pdf. Accessed May 28, 2020.

Enhanced Recovery After Surgery
An Update of the Current Standard of Surgical Care

Erin L. Sherer, EdD, PA-C, RD[a],*, Elizabeth C. Erickson, MS, PA-C[b],
Margaret H. Holland, MSHS, PA-C[c]

KEYWORDS

- Enhanced recovery after surgery • ERAS • Protocol

KEY POINTS

- Enhanced recovery after surgery (ERAS) is an evidence-based approach to surgical care that attempts to reduce the stress of surgery and encourages a quick return to the patient's normal life.
- ERAS protocols can help improve clinical outcomes by reducing length-of-stay, reducing postoperative complications, and providing cost savings (for both hospital and patient).
- Successful ERAS protocols are dependent on multidisciplinary team approaches to care, support from hospital administration, and continued auditing to improve processes.
- Research to improve patient outcomes after surgery is ongoing. Current protocols frequently are revised and new ones are being developed for surgical specialties.

INTRODUCTION

Imagine a world in which patients recover quickly from surgery with few to no complications. That was the vision surgeons had for their patients when they began developing the enhanced recovery after surgery (ERAS) protocols.[1] In 1999, a group of Danish surgeons led by Dr Henrik Kehlet, described a perioperative care program for patients that helped encourage early ambulation and reduce hospital length of stay after colorectal surgery.[2] This landmark study introduced the fast-track concept in surgery. This theory suggested that if patients followed a standardized, multimodal approach to rehabilitation and care, they would have improved outcomes.[2–4]

[a] Emergency Department, Columbia University Irving Medical Center, 622 West 168th Street, New York, NY 10032, USA; [b] MidMichigan Medical Center, 4201 Campus Ridge Drive, Suite 2000, Midland, MI 48640, USA; [c] Department of Cardiac Surgery, Boston Children's Hospital, 300 Longwood Avenue, Bader 273, Boston, MA 02115, USA
* Corresponding author.
E-mail address: els2183@cumc.columbia.edu

Physician Assist Clin 6 (2021) 267–279
https://doi.org/10.1016/j.cpha.2020.11.002
2405-7991/21/© 2020 Elsevier Inc. All rights reserved.

Based on Dr Kehlet's fast-track concept, European surgeons were able to develop the first ERAS protocols. In developing these protocols, the group's primary focus was to improve surgical recovery and reduce complications by "modifying the metabolic response to surgical insult rather than just limiting the length of stay."[1]

Although ERAS protocols were initiated in 2001, there still was minimal change across most health care systems.[1] The ERAS Society, an international nonprofit organization composed of clinicians, was created to "develop perioperative care and to improve recovery through research, education, audit and implementation of evidence-based practice."[5,6] Interest in ERAS has grown since its inception, and researchers have continued to investigate and improve on this approach to care. At the time of this writing, there are 17 ERAS Society Consensus Guidelines that have been published, and it is likely that more will be developed in the future (**Table 1**).

WHY WAS ENHANCED RECOVERY AFTER SURGERY DEVELOPED?

Part of the difficulty in caring for surgical patients is that the process often involves multiple steps and professionals that can have an impact on the quality of care. For example, a patient initially may be seen by an outpatient health care provider and then an inpatient provider for preoperative care, the surgical team, the postoperative recovery team, and even a different clinician or team for postsurgical follow-up. Each care provider, each facility, and each interaction the patient has effects on the others.

ERAS was developed in an attempt to try to standardize and improve patient care throughout a patient's surgical journey.[1] The protocols allow for the different

Table 1
Enhanced recovery after surgery society guidelines

Procedure or Specialty	Year of Publication (or Latest Revision)
Cesarean delivery	2019
Hip and knee replacement	2019
Cardiac surgery	2019
Lung surgery	2019
Gynecologic oncology	2019
Colorectal surgery	2018
Esophagectomy	2018
Head and neck cancer surgery	2017
Breast reconstructive surgery	2017
Bariatric surgery	2016
Liver surgery	2016
Gastrointestinal surgery	2015
Gastrectomy	2014
Radical cystectomy for bladder cancer	2013
Pancreaticoduodenectomy	2012
Rectal/pelvic surgery	2012
Elective colonic surgery	2012

Adapted from the ERAS Society. https://erassociety.org/. Published 2016. Accessed on February 29, 2020.

departments and health care providers to work together to improve outcomes and a faster return to normalcy for the patient. There are several key components to the ERAS protocols: a multidisciplinary team working together around the patient; a multimodal approach to resolving issues that delay recovery and cause complications; a scientific, evidence-based approach to care protocols; and a change in management using an interactive and continuous auditing system.[1]

COMPONENTS OF ENHANCED RECOVERY AFTER SURGERY

ERAS relies on the belief that single element by itself improves outcomes of surgery—each process has an impact on the next.[1] Therefore, it is imperative that the components of care are harmonious. Many health care providers are involved in the care of the surgical patient and each must work together to agree on the end points of management in order for the protocol to be successful.[1] The surgeon and the anesthesiologist usually are the medical leaders of the protocol.[1] There usually is an ERAS project manager (often a nurse) who is responsible for facilitating the resources and management to introduce the protocols.[1] There also an is ERAS coordinator (often an advanced practice provider) who manages practical matters, such as composing and distributing memos and instructions, managing feedback to the units, and arranging for continuous training of new personnel.[1] In addition to creating the ERAS team, it is important that each person understands their role, including the patient (Fig. 1).[7] In some instances, a champion, or dedicated team member, is tasked with helping

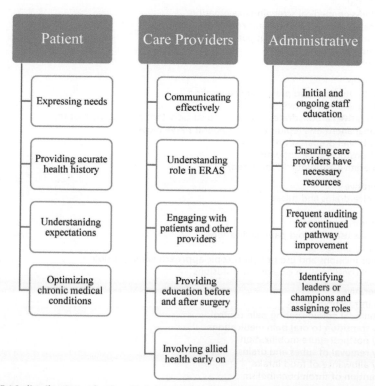

Fig. 1. ERAS distribution of roles. (*Adapted from* the American Association of Nurse Anesthetists. https://www.aana.com/practice/clinical-practice-resources/enhanced-recovery-after-surgery. Published 2019. Accessed on February 29, 2020.)

everyone understand their individual roles. It also is important and necessary that other clinicians participate in the protocol to support its success—these include occupational therapists, registered dietitians, and physical therapists.[1,8]

A typical ERAS protocol includes 20 or more core elements of care that are evidence based (**Box 1**).[5,6] Usually these elements are broken down into 4 main categories: preadmission, preoperative, intraoperative, and postoperative.[5,6] A majority of these elements focus on reducing stress and improving the body's response to surgical stress and the idea of prehabilitation before surgery.[6] A critical element of ERAS that sometimes is overlooked in protocols is the goal of improving a patient's physical health, before surgery even begins.

PREADMISSION

Preadmission elements of ERAS typically begin with the patient and the primary care provider (PCP).[6,7] A complete history and physical examination should be performed to review all comorbid conditions and to highlight any uncontrolled medical conditions.[9] For example, a chronic medical condition like uncontrolled diabetes should be optimized prior to surgery, because poorly controlled diabetics are at high risk

---

Box 1
General enhanced recovery after surgery components

Preadmission
  Preadmission medical screening examination
  Medical optimization of chronic conditions
  Nutritional counseling and support
  Cessation of smoking
  Control alcohol intake

Preoperative
  Patient education and presurgery counseling
  Meeting with care providers
  Preoperative carbohydrate drink prior to surgery (not nothing by mouth)
  Regional anesthesia (epidural or peripheral nerve block)
  Select bowel prepartation
  Select postoperative antiemetic
  Preoperative antibiotic (if indicated)

Perioperative
  Minimize drains and tubes
  GDFT
  Temperature control
  Judicious use of opioid pain medications
  Regional analgesia
  Shorter incisions and use of laparoscopic approach when possible
  Careful consideration of blood transfusions

Postoperative
  Stop intravenous fluids
  Multimodal opioid-sparing pain control
  Early transition to oral pain medications
  Early postprocedure mobilization
  Early removal of tubes and drains
  Early allowance of food intake
  Prevention of thromboembolism

Adapted from the ERAS Society. https://erassociety.org/. Published 2016. Accessed on February 29, 2020.

for postoperative complications.[10] ERAS guidelines also suggest that patients should discontinue smoking and alcohol use 4 weeks before surgery.[11] The patient's PCP can encourage the patient to follow these guidelines and may prescribe medications to help, if necessary.

PREOPERATIVE

Preoperative ERAS considerations focus on patient education, approach to diet, pain control, antiemetic initiation, and bowel preparation.[5] Patient education and appropriate counseling are necessary for ERAS to be successful.[7,9] The patient should be provided with literature (at the appropriate reading level) and verbal education about the surgery and the postoperative period, in order to discuss potential complications and set proper expectations for recovery.[9]

Recommendations for preoperative nutrition have changed over the years. In the past, many patients were told to eat nothing after midnight before surgery. Research shows, however, that carbohydrate loading before surgery increases insulin sensitivity, decreases postoperative inflammation, and decreases length of hospital stay.[12,13] The ERAS guidelines suggest patients should stop eating solid food 6 hours before surgery and clear fluids 2 hours before surgery.[14,15]

Providers may implement strategies to manage postsurgical pain in the preoperative period. ERAS protocols typically recommend a multimodal approach using non-narcotic pain management methods, such as oral pregabalin, gabapentin, and acetaminophen. Nonsteroidal anti-inflammatory drugs (NSAIDs) also may be used; however, some studies have shown an increased risk for anastomotic leaks in colorectal resections and they should be used with caution.[16] Additionally, neuraxial and field blocks can help reduce the use of intraoperative and postoperative opioid use.[9] The selection of preoperative medication may vary; there is no standard combination. Medication selection often is dependent on the medication formulary of the hospital and preferences of the surgical and/or anesthesia team.

ERAS protocols also encourage the prevention of postoperative nausea and vomiting through the use of antiemetics and corticosteroids. For example, dexamethasone may be administered preoperatively to prevent nausea and decrease the perioperative stress response.[9] Antiemetic prophylaxis should be administered in the operating room, prior to extubation.[9]

In the past, patients were instructed to perform a mechanical bowel preparation before surgery.[17] Current ERAS Society guidelines recommend against this practice. Evidence indicates there is no impact on morbidity or mortality in patients when mechanical bowel preparation is used compared with no bowel preparation or rectal enema alone.[5] Some evidence suggests that bowel preparation, when combined with oral antibiotics, decreases the rate of surgical site infections (SSIs) patients undergoing colorectal surgery; however, there currently are no recommendations to use antibiotics solely for this purpose.[17]

PERIOPERATIVE

ERAS recommendations for the perioperative period include minimizing drains and tubes, managing fluids carefully, controlling body temperature, using pain control cautiously, using regional analgesia when appropriate, creating small incisions or using laparoscopic approaches when possible, and carefully considering blood transfusions.[5]

The use of drains and tubes has been a common practice during surgery, but ERAS protocols now recommend limited use or no use of these at all, depending on the type of surgery performed.[18–20] Historically, surgeons have placed drains (for example a Jackson-Pratt or chest tube) for monitoring of fluid or air postoperatively.[21–23] Evidence indicates, however, these drains may cause more harm than benefit in pancreatic, colonic, hepatic, and gynecologic surgery because they do not improve overall patient outcomes.[18,19,22,24,25] Additionally, the use of nasogastric intubation is not recommended because it can lead to an increased risk of postoperative pneumonia.[21,22] Urinary catheters often are used during surgeries because procedures sometimes can be lengthy and surgeons want to monitor urine output, but ERAS recommendations indicate that if these are used, they need to be removed early to prevent catheter-associated urinary tract infections.[19,21] Limiting the use of drains and tubes also reduces the need for pain medication related to the drains and supports early ambulation.[21]

Fluid management during the perioperative period is paramount to the success of ERAS. Although maintaining euvolemia, or optimal fluid balance, during surgery can be difficult, providing inadequate fluids during surgery can be harmful.[6] Goal-directed fluid therapy (GDFT) is recommended to prevent overhydrating or underhydrating surgical patients, because it can decrease morbidity, mortality, and health care costs.[6,9] GDFT involves cardiovascular monitoring to determine the need for additional fluid, vasopressors, or inotropes during surgery.[6] Serum brain natriuretic peptide levels also can assess accurately intravascular volume status in surgical patients.[9]

Techniques to control body temperature, specifically aimed at maintaining normothermia (a temperature between 36°C and 38°C), are part of ERAS. Intraoperative hypothermia has been associated with higher risks of SSIs and cardiac events.[6,23,24] Hypothermia may occur during surgery because anesthesia has an impact on the thermoregulatory system, the skin surface is exposed to a cold environment, and cold intravenous fluids are used.[6,24] Research indicates that intraoperative warming can reduce SSIs, cardiovascular complications, and surgical blood loss.[26] Normothermia can be achieved by increasing the ambient room temperature and using systemic warming devices, forced air warming blankets, and warmed intravenous fluids.[6]

Efforts to control pain perioperatively should focus on using regional analgesia when appropriate. ERAS supports a multimodal approach to pain control in an effort to decrease the use of opioids.[9,25] Opioids have adverse effects, such as nausea, vomiting, sedation, ileus, and respiratory depression—all of which can have an impact on a patient's ability to recover quickly after surgery.[25] Avoiding the use of opioids may be possible if alternative medications are used or if spinal analgesia/transverse abdominis plane blocks are initiated preoperatively.[25] Alternative perioperative pain control medications include lidocaine infusions, α_2-agonists like dexmedetomidine, ketamine, magnesium sulfate, high-dose steroids, and gabapentinoids.[25]

ERAS protocols recommend that surgical incisions are small and that minimally invasive surgical approaches be used (when possible). Using minimally invasive techniques reduces the trauma and immunologic impact of surgery compared with open approaches.[25] Laparoscopic versus open surgery for colorectal cancer reduces recovery time, length of stay, blood loss, and complications.[25] Minimally invasive approaches also support other aspects of ERAS, such as reducing the need for pain medication, supporting early ambulation, reducing fluid shifts, and reducing ileus formation.[25]

To enhance surgical recovery and reduce complications, it is imperative that providers try to avoid (or carefully consider) the use of perioperative blood products.[25] Providing blood products perioperatively may have an impact on long-term survival in surgical patients.[25,27,28] It is essential that providers try to correct anemia preoperatively, to prevent the need for blood transfusion during surgery. Intravenous iron should be considered as an alternative for correcting abnormalities and preventing the use of blood products.[25,29]

POSTOPERATIVE

ERAS protocols for postoperative care are designed to support a quick recovery. Ideally, a patient following an ERAS protocol should be drinking, eating, mobilizing, and sleeping on the day after an operation.[1] Postoperative ERAS protocols typically focus on discontinuing intravenous fluids, using multimodal pain control, removing tubes and drains as quickly as possible, and initiating oral intake early.[1,5,6,9]

As discussed previously, maintaining a euvolemic state is beneficial to the patient because it can decrease morbidity, mortality, and health care costs.[6,9] If the patient is tolerating oral intake, it is reasonable to stop intravenous fluids within 24 hours of surgery to avoid fluid overload.[6] This also can aid the patient in early mobilization.[6]

In the postoperative period, ERAS protocols support narcotic-sparing approaches to pain control. Opiate analgesia has many side effects, such as postoperative ileus, constipation, nausea, drowsiness, confusion, and respiratory depression.[6] All of these side effects can have an impact on a patient's ability to recover quickly. ERAS protocols typically support early introduction of oral pain medications, such as acetaminophen, NSAIDs, and gabapentinoids in the postoperative period.[6,9] Some patients and procedures, however, are more complicated than others, and each situation should be assessed individually.

There are benefits to initiating oral intake early. Most patients who begin oral feeding early regain bowel function faster, have a shorter length of stay in the hospital, and have decreased complications.[30] Early oral intake usually means the patient receives food within 24 hours of surgery, starting with clear fluids and advancing to the standard diet as tolerated.[6]

Efforts also should be aimed at reducing postoperative nausea and vomiting with antiemetics and opioid avoidance, because these can be barriers to early mobilization and oral intake.[6] In addition to oral intake, chewing gum sometimes is incorporated into ERAS protocols. Chewing gum postoperatively decreases time to first flatus and first bowel movement, making it a relatively easy and low-risk intervention to implement.[6] Postoperative laxatives (such as magnesium hydroxide and bisacodyl) may be a part ERAS protocols because they can help reduce the time and discomfort associated with the first postoperative bowel movement.[6]

A critical part of ERAS is early mobilization. Early postoperative ambulation and movement help prevent pulmonary complications, loss of skeletal muscle, thromboembolic complications, and insulin resistance and decreases ileus.[6,25] Patients following ERAS protocols should try to ambulate within 24 hours of surgery, although this can depend on the type of surgery and the individual patient. Most ERAS protocols suggest the patient should be mobilizing for at least 2 hours on the day of surgery, followed by 6 hours every day after.[6] It is important to recognize that aggressive early mobilization likely requires the help and support of the entire health care team.

Prevention of venous thromboembolism also is a critical postoperative consideration that is included in some ERAS protocols. A combination of mechanical compression and medication (such as heparin, low-molecular-weight heparin, and direct oral anticoagulants) typically is initiated in the intraoperative or immediate postoperative period for prophylaxis.[6,25] Extended prophylaxis for 28 days should be considered, depending on a patient's medical comorbidities and history as well as the type of surgery.[6] It is recommended that clinicians use decision-making tools, such as the Caprini risk score calculator, to help stratify risk and determine which patients may benefit from extended thromboprophylaxis.[31]

Finally, it is important to remove tubes and drains as quickly as possible to reduce rates of infection and to encourage patients to ambulate early.[6] ERAS protocols suggest urinary catheter removal within the first 24 hours of surgery, if not intraoperatively.[6] To facilitate this, cutoffs for urinary output typically range from 20 mL to 30 mL of urine per hour before the catheter is removed.[6] Early urinary catheter removal in patients with epidural analgesia is feasible and has no long-term complications.[20] Nasogastric/orogastric tubes should be removed before reversal of anesthesia or as soon as possible.[25]

BENEFITS OF ENHANCED RECOVERY AFTER SURGERY

There are many well-documented benefits of ERAS.[6,32–34] One of the most notable successes of ERAS is the reduction in rates of surgical complications. For example, a meta-analysis of 16 randomized trials examining postoperative morbidity in colorectal surgery patients found a reduction in complications by 40% (relative risk [RR] 0.6; 95% CI, 0.46–0.76).[33] Another meta-analysis of 39 trials found a significant decrease in complication rates (odds ratio [OR] 0.70; 95% CI, 0.56–0.86; $P = .001$) for noncolorectal surgery patients treated in ERAS programs.[34]

To reduce complications, however, care providers and patients must adhere to the protocols. A study published in the *Journal of the American Medical Association* in 2019 indicated there is a direct correlation between reduced complication rates and high compliance with ERAS protocols.[35] The Postoperative Outcomes Within Enhanced Recovery After Surgery Protocol (POWER) study evaluated outcomes between elective colorectal surgery patients who either followed ERAS protocols or did not follow a protocol. The prospective cohort study included 2084 adult patients in multiple centers over a 4-month period in 2017.[35] The study found that the number of patients with moderate or severe complications was lower in the ERAS group (25.2% vs 30.3%, respectively; OR 0.77; 95% CI, 0.63–0.94; $P = .01$) and that adherence to ERAS protocol was 63.6% (interquartile range, 54.5%–77.3%).[35] The investigators concluded that an increase in ERAS compliance was associated with decreased postoperative complications.[35]

A follow up study entitled POWER2, confirmed these findings to be true in orthopedic surgery as well.[36] The POWER2 study assessed the association of the use of ERAS protocols with complications in patients undergoing elective total hip arthroplasty (THA) and total knee arthroplasty (TKA).[36] The multicenter, prospective, cohort study included 6146 adult patients who underwent elective THA or TKA during a 2-month period in 2018.[36] Patients with high adherence to ERAS protocols had fewer overall postoperative complications (144 [10.6%] vs 270 [13.0%], respectively; OR 0.80; 95% CI, 0.64–0.99; $P<.001$).[36]

ERAS protocols also have reduced the length of stay in hospitals and produced a cost savings benefit. A reduction in length of stay was a major finding from a large trial in the United Kingdom, including 16,267 surgical patients from 72 hospital sites in from 2009 to 2012.[37] The study examined length of stay and compliance with each element of the ERAS protocols for colorectal, orthopedic, urologic, and gynecologic surgery.[37] The researchers found that ERAS compliance rates of greater than 80% were associated with a statistically significant shorter length of stay in all specialties except gynecology (P = .0796).[37] The investigators concluded that compliance with ERAS is associated with a shorter median length of stay, which represents a clinically important reduction in morbidity and significant cost-savings.[37]

Decreasing complications and lengths of stay lead to financial benefits as well. Several studies have identified cost savings when ERAS protocols are implemented.[34,38–41] For example, researchers found that in colorectal and gynecologic surgery, implementing an ERAS protocol led to average savings of $2200 to $2500 per patient.[39] A study involving only gynecology patients found that ERAS protocols reduced the overall costs per patient by $4381.[40] Lastly, a recent meta-analysis found that ERAS protocols in noncolorectal surgery presented a per-patient cost savings of $5109.10 (95% CI, $4365.80–$5852.40; P<.001).[34]

Even though it is costly to implement an ERAS protocol, a study in the United States found it provides a significant return on investment.[38] The investigators of the study indicated that it costs $552,783 to implement an ERAS program; however, this was offset by a savings of nearly $948,500 in the first year (net savings of $395,717).[38] Researchers in Alberta, Canada, found ERAS programs to be cost-effective as well.[41] They found that for every $1 invested in the ERAS protocol, there was a savings of $3.8 (range of $2.8–$5.1).[41]

IMPLEMENTATION AND SUSTAINABILITY OF ENHANCED RECOVERY AFTER SURGERY

There are many potential barriers to the implementation of ERAS. Research has indicated that education and training for clinicians in ERAS are insufficient.[1] One reason for this may be that it may take time for clinicians and hospitals to understand the impact of new data and to implement change. Clinical practice often does not change until approximately 15 years after there is clear evidence indicating there is significant value in changing behavior.[42] Therefore, it is important that clinicians be educated properly about the benefits of ERAS. Other barriers to implementation of ERAS protocols include general resistance to change, lack of time and staff, and poor communication, collaboration, and coordination between departments.[1,43] Additionally, managers may be reluctant to invest in ERAS programs because of the initial cost.[1]

Once an ERAS protocol is in place, auditing is an important part of how successful it will be. The care process is complex and this can lead to confusion and misunderstanding about goals and outcomes.[1] By continuous auditing of the care process, clinicians can gain a better understanding of the successes and failures of their program. Health care professionals often believe their patient care outcomes are better than they actually are, that surgical team compliance is higher than it actually is, and that hospital stays are shorter than they actually are.[1,8] The ERAS Society has developed an audit system to assist in reviewing and improving an institution's protocol.

Sustainability is key to the success of the enhanced recovery program.[44] For this reason, the ERAS society has developed a program to help improve education and compliance. Most hospital programs that have shown sustained improvements in new protocols include a workplace culture that is open to change, the formation of teams that work to improve communication and collaboration, the support of hospital management, and the use of standardized order sets to encourage use.[43,45]

SUMMARY

Evidence-based ERAS protocols provide a consistent approach to surgical care for all patients, regardless of the location or health care provider. Because ERAS principles are applied across all surgical specialties, researchers and management teams must continue to innovate, audit, and improve these processes. New and revised procedure-specific consensus guidelines will help improve outcomes in all specialties.[1]

Implementation of an ERAS protocol can be challenging, but the advantages for patients and potential savings for the health care system are worth the effort. Successful programs require the participation and education of the entire medical staff and the patients. Long-term success of ERAS programs will depend on continued improvements in care processes, protocols, auditing, and feedback. ERAS protocols will continue to be an important part of the health care model as patient outcomes, quality measures, and cost reduction become more important to stakeholders and patients.

CLINICS CARE POINTS

- Protocols can help guide care, but every surgical patient is different and will require a tailored multi-disciplinary approach to treatment.
- Care providers all need to work together for ERAS protocols to be implemented effectively.
- Early patient education and communication are key to implementing ERAS protocols and improving surgical outcomes.
- Multimodal approaches to pain management can help reduce the need for opioids following surgery.
- Physician assistants have an important role in improving patient care outcomes using ERAS protocols in all components of the surgical process.

DISCLOSURE

The authors have nothing to disclose.

REFERENCES

1. Ljungqvist O, Scott M, Fearon KC. Enhanced Recovery After Surgery: A Review. JAMA Surg 2017;152(3):292–8.
2. Kehlet H, Mogensen T. Hospital stay of 2 days after open sigmoidectomy with a multimodal rehabilitation programme. Br J Surg 1999;86(2):227–30.
3. Delaney CP, Fazio VW, Senagore AJ, et al. 'Fast track' postoperative management protocol for patients with high co-morbidity undergoing complex abdominal and pelvic colorectal surgery. Br J Surg 2001;88(11):1533–8.
4. Schilling PL, Dimick JB, Birkmeyer JD. Prioritizing quality improvement in general surgery. J Am Coll Surg 2008;207:698–704.
5. ERAS Society. 2016. Available at: https://erassociety.org/. Accessed February 29, 2020.
6. Altman AD, Helpman L, McGee J, et al. Enhanced recovery after surgery: implementing a new standard of surgical care. CAMJ 2019;191(17):E469–75.
7. Hughes M, Coolsen MME, Aahlin EK, et al. Attitudes of patients and care providers to enhanced recovery after surgery programs after major abdominal surgery. J Surg Res 2015;193:102–10.
8. Gotlib Conn L, McKenzie M, Pearsall EA, et al. Successful implementation of an enhanced recovery after surgery programme for elective colorectal surgery: a process evaluation of champions' experiences. Implement Sci 2015;10:99.
9. Kim BJ, Aloia TA. What is "enhanced recovery," and how can I do it? J Gastrointest Surg 2018;22(1):164–71.

10. Kim BJ, Tzeng CD, Cooper AB, et al. Borderline operability in hepatectomy patients is associated with higher rates of failure to rescue after severe complications. J Surg Oncol 2017;115(3):337–43.

11. Nelson G, Altman AD, Nick A, et al. Guidelines for pre- and intra-operative care in gynecologic/oncology surgery: Enhanced Recovery after Surgery (ERAS®) Society recommendations — part 1. Gynecol Oncol 2016;140:313–22.

12. Smith MD, McCall J, Plank L, et al. Preoperative carbohydrate treatment for enhancing recovery after elective surgery. Cochrane Database Syst Rev 2014; 8. https://doi.org/10.1002/14651858.

13. Webster J, Osborne SR, Gill R, et al. Does preoperative oral carbohydrate reduce hospital stay? A randomized trial. AORN J 2014;99:233–42.

14. Practice guidelines for preoperative fasting and the use of pharmacologic agents to reduce the risk of pulmonary aspiration: application to healthy patients undergoing elective procedures: an updated report by the American Society of Anesthesiologists Task Force on Preoperative Fasting and the Use of Pharmacologic Agents to Reduce the Risk of Pulmonary Aspiration. Anesthesiology 2017;126: 376–93.

15. Smith I, Kranke P, Murat I, et al. Perioperative fasting in adults and children: guidelines from the European Society of Anaesthesiology. Eur J Anaesthesiol 2011;28:556–69.

16. Subendran J, Siddiqui N, Victor JC, et al. NSAID use and anastomotic leaks following elective colorectal surgery: a matched case-control study. J Gastrointest Surg 2014;18:1391–7.

17. Yamada T, Yokoyama Y, Takeda K, et al. Preoperative bowel preparation in ERAS Program: would-be merits or demerits. In: Fukushima R, Kailborim, editors. Enhanced recovery after surgery. Singapore: Springer; 2018. p. 21–7.

18. Abeles A, Kwasnicki RM, Darzi A. Enhanced recovery after surgery: current research insights and future direction. World J Gastrointest Surg 2017;9(2): 37–45.

19. van Woerden V, Wong-Lun-hing E, Lodewick T, et al. Abandoning prophylactic abdominal drainage after hepatic surgery: 10 years of no-drain policy in an ERAS environment. HPB (Oxford) 2019;21:S572–3.

20. Schreiber A, Aydil E, Walschus U, et al. Early removal of urinary drainage in patients receiving epidural analgesia after colorectal surgery within an ERAS protocol is feasible. Langenbecks Arch Surg 2019;404:853–63.

21. Cheatham ML, Chapman WC, Key SP, et al. A meta-analysis of selective versus routine nasogastric decompression after elective laparotomy. Ann Surg 1995; 221:469–76 [discussion: 476–8].

22. Petrowsky H, Demartines N, Rousson V, et al. Evidence-based value of prophylactic drainage in gastrointestinal surgery: a systematic review and meta-analyses. Ann Surg 2004;240:1074–84 [discussion: 1084–5].

23. Wong PF, Kumar S, Bohra A, et al. Randomized clinical trial of perioperative systemic warming in major elective abdominal surgery. Br J Surg 2007;94:421–6.

24. Nelson G, Bakkum-Gamez J, Kalogera E, et al. Guidelines for perioperative care in gynecologic/oncology: Enhanced Recovery After Surgery (ERAS) Society recommendations—2019 update. Int J Gynecol Cancer 2019;29:651–68.

25. Gustafsson UO, Scott MJ, Hubner M, et al. Guidelines for perioperative care in elective colorectal surgery: enhanced recovery after surgery (ERAS) Society Recommendations: 2018. World J Surg 2019;43:659–95.

26. Madrid E, Urrútia G, Roqué i Figuls M, et al. Active body surface warming systems for preventing complications caused by inadvertent perioperative hypothermia in adults. Cochrane Database Syst Rev 2016;(4):CD009016.

27. Acheson AG, Brookes MJ, Spahn DR. Effects of allogeneic red blood cell transfusions on clinical outcomes in patients undergoing colorectal cancer surgery: a systematic review and meta-analysis. Ann Surg 2012;256:235–44.

28. Smilowitz NR, Oberweis BS, Nukala S, et al. Association between anemia, bleeding, and transfusion with long-term mortality following noncardiac surgery. Am J Med 2016;129:315–23.

29. Shin HW, Park JJ, Kim HJ, et al. Efficacy of perioperative intravenous iron therapy for transfusion in orthopedic surgery: A systematic review and meta-analysis. PLoS One 2019;14(5):e0215427.

30. Minig L, Biffi R, Zanagnolo V, et al. Early oral versus "traditional" postoperative feeding in gynecologic oncology patients undergoing intestinal resection: a randomized controlled trial. Ann Surg Oncol 2009;16:1660–8.

31. Bell BR, Bastien PE, Douketis JD. Thrombosis Canada. Prevention of venous thromboembolism in the Enhanced Recovery After Surgery (ERAS) setting: an evidence-based review. Can J Anaesth 2015;62:194–202.

32. Lau CSM, Chamberlain RS. Enhanced recovery after surgery programs improve patient outcomes and recovery: a meta-analysis. World J Surg 2017;41:899–913.

33. Greco M, Capretti G, Beretta L, et al. Enhanced recovery program in colorectal surgery: a meta-analysis of randomized controlled trials. World J Surg 2014;38(6):1531–41.

34. Visioni A, Shah R, Gabriel E, et al. Enhanced recovery after surgery for noncolorectal surgery?: a systematic review and meta-analysis of major abdominal surgery. Ann Surg 2018;267(1):57–65.

35. Ripollés-Melchor J, Ramírez-Rodríguez JM, Casans-Francés R, et al. Association between use of enhanced recovery after surgery protocol and postoperative complications in colorectal surgery: the postoperative outcomes within enhanced recovery after surgery protocol (POWER) study. JAMA Surg 2019;154(8):725–36.

36. Ripollés-Melchor J, Abad-Motos A, Díez-Remesal Y, et al. Association between use of enhanced recovery after surgery protocol and postoperative complications in total hip and knee arthroplasty in the postoperative outcomes within enhanced recovery after surgery protocol in elective total hip and knee arthroplasty study (POWER2). JAMA Surg 2020. https://doi.org/10.1001/jamasurg.2019.6024.

37. Simpson JC, Moonesinghe SR, Grocott MP, et al. National Enhanced Recovery Partnership Advisory Board. Enhanced recovery from surgery in the UK: an audit of the enhanced recovery partnership programme 2009–2012. Br J Anaesth 2015;115(4):560–8.

38. Stone AB, Grant MC, Roda CP, et al. Implementation costs of an enhanced recovery after surgery program in the United States: a financial model and sensitivity analysis based on experiences at a quaternary academic medical center. J Am Coll Surg 2016;222(3):219–25.

39. Mendivil AA, Busch JR, Richards DC, et al. The Impact of an enhanced recovery after surgery program on patients treated for gynecologic cancer in the community hospital setting. Int J Gynecol Cancer 2018;28:581–5.

40. Pache B, Joliat GR, Hübner M, et al. Cost-analysis of enhanced recovery after surgery (ERAS) program in gynecologic surgery. Gynecol Oncol 2019;154:388–93.

41. Thanh NX, Chuck AW, Wasylak T, et al. An economic evaluation of the Enhanced Recovery After Surgery (ERAS) multisite implementation program for colorectal surgery in Alberta. Can J Surg 2016;59:415–21.
42. Lassen K, Hannemann P, Ljungqvist O, et al. Enhanced Recovery After Surgery Group. Patterns in current perioperative practice: survey of colorectal surgeons in five northern European countries. BMJ 2005;330(7505):1420–1.
43. Pearsall EA, Meghji Z, Pitzul KB, et al. A qualitative study to understand the barriers and enablers in implementing an enhanced recovery after surgery program. Ann Surg 2015;261(1):92–6.
44. Roulin D, Donadini A, Gander S, et al. Cost-effectiveness of the implementation of an enhanced recovery protocol for colorectal surgery. Br J Surg 2013;100(8): 1108–14.
45. Ament SM, Gillissen F, Moser A, et al. Identification of promising strategies to sustain improvements in hospital practice: a qualitative case study. BMC Health Serv Res 2014;14(1):641.

Disaster Surgery

Mary Showstark, MPAS, PA-C

KEYWORDS

- Disaster medicine • Austere medicine • Mass casualty incident • Surgery
- Physician assistant

KEY POINTS

- Surgery in times of disaster.
- Working with limited resources.
- Sterilization in times of disaster.
- Ethical standards in surgery in disaster.

INTRODUCTION

Disaster surgery historically has had the notion of being related to the military. Surgeons, corpsmen, and parajumpers performing damage control surgery and stabilizing patients for transport to a receiving hospital is what comes to mind.[1] Although this topic relates highly to the military and war, it is becoming common place in everyday society, as disasters can strike in a moment's notice. With the increasing global surface temperatures, more heat in the atmosphere, warm ocean, and rising sea levels, the world is at risk for more natural disasters. Few disasters are pre-warned. These include hurricanes and severe storms. Other natural disasters with minimal to no warning include floods, tsunamis, tornadoes, wildfires, landslides, droughts, earthquakes, and volcanic eruptions. Chemical and nuclear disasters can occur, and urban centers around the world are being plagued with terror attacks and mass shootings. Disasters, no matter the type, can affect and overwhelm a hospital system and a community quickly. This article discusses disaster surgery as it pertains to environmental and man-made disasters and the role of the physician assistant in disaster surgery.

SEQUENCE OF EVENTS AFTER A LARGE-SCALE ENVIRONMENTAL DISASTER

There are usually several simultaneous pieces that happen after a disaster. First the media arrives on scene. The next thing that happens is nongovernmental organizations (NGOs) and foreign medical teams begin to mobilize. Different organizations

Yale University School of Medicine, Physician Assistant Online Program, 100 Church Street South, Suite A230, New Haven, CT 06519, USA
E-mail address: mary.showstark@yale.edu

Physician Assist Clin 6 (2021) 281–294
https://doi.org/10.1016/j.cpha.2020.11.007
2405-7991/21/© 2020 Elsevier Inc. All rights reserved.

begin to enter the disaster zone, including federal, state, and tribal that perform an assessment of the area and measure damage and the needs of the community. Agencies begin to mobilize at the command of federal orders on the State's request for aid. An Emergency Operations Plan (EOP) and an Emergency Operations Center (EOC) are created. All agencies begin to work through this system in a chain of command, known as the Incident Command System (ICS), with the EOC as a command center; however, other organizations that will create their own base of operations and have their own command centers, all should report to the EOC[2,3] (**Fig. 1**). The ICS is an adaptable system built around Incident Command, Operations, Planning, Logistics, and Finance/Administration.[4] Although all teams are required to report to the EOC, Federal Emergency Management Agency (FEMA), World Health Organization/Pan American Health Organization (WHO/PAHO), less than 25% of teams followed these protocols after disasters such as what occurred in the Haiti 2010 earthquake.[5] Because of this lack of communication, duplication of efforts and lack of resource utilization tend to ensue in many disaster settings.

Nevertheless, multiple federal and state agencies descend on the scene. Search and rescue teams begin their missions and agencies such as FEMA, Red Cross, Drug Enforcement Administration (DEA), Department of Agriculture, Small Business Association, and Wildlife and Gaming. Medical teams such as Disaster Medical Assistance Teams (DMAT) and International Medical/Surgical Response Teams (IMSuRT) who may have been pre-staged in a nearby area begin to deploy to create field hospitals or work out of existing structures (**Fig. 2**). Logistics, Operations, Supplies, Security, Medical, Air Operations (Ops), Strike Teams, Food Units, Communications, Legal, Infectious Disease, Women's Health, lesbian, gay, bisexual, transgender, transsexual, queer (LGBTTQ) Health, Water Sanitation and Hygiene (WaSH), and Petrol, Shipping Mitigation experts also arrive. Evacuations, shelters, and makeshift hospitals begin. Sometimes hospitals will still be open but may not be functional creating surges into nearby hospitals. Multiple patients will begin to arrive on scene if a makeshift hospital has been set up. In the London Bombings and Tokyo Sarin attacks in the subways, ambulances became overwhelmed and people used any available transport to reach the hospitals.[6] For this reason, many times, makeshift hospitals are set up nearby or in the parking lot of the hospital or near an accessible area such as an airport tarmac as in the case in Grand Bahama after Hurricane Dorian and the 2010 Haiti Earthquake. After the 2004 Tsunami in Thailand, more than 1400 operations were

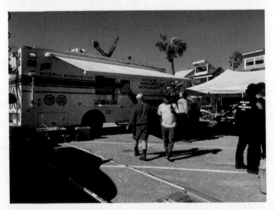

Fig. 1. Base of operations: USAR, office of emergency management mobile setup: Mexico beach, Florida: Hurricane Michael.

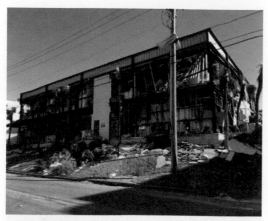

Fig. 2. Existing hospital in Panama City, Florida: Hurricane Michael. Parts of the hospital were still functioning.

performed in the first 3 days using emergency rooms as makeshift operating areas and having supplies and staff airlifted into the disaster zone.[7]

TRIAGE IN ALL TYPES OF DISASTER

Triage begins and patients are evacuated to the nearest hospital. Sometimes this is not possible. Sometimes an area is so badly affected that the potential for multiple patients is too great and field hospitals are set up. Field hospitals or clinics may consist of a make-shift tarp (**Fig. 3**) or it may be dome tents donated by agencies such as Cirque de Soleil (**Figs. 4** and **5**) in Haiti or more military grade such as Western Shelter tents (**Fig. 6**). The decision to set up a field hospital depends on many factors such as the ability to evacuate, the amount of people that live in the affected area, the social vulnerability of the population, the access to the nearest functioning hospital, the knowledge of another imminent disaster, and the ability of the hospitals in the area to reopen and function.

When multiple patients arrive on scene, triage is a necessity. Maximum benefit for the maximum number of patients in the shortest time with the available resources is the key to triage.[4] Labeling a patient as more critical than they actually are happens

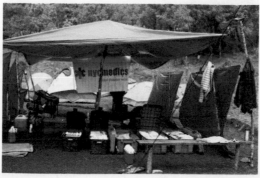

Fig. 3. Medical tent setup using tarps in remote village of Nepal: Earthquake 2015.

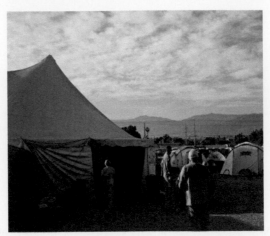

Fig. 4. Field hospital: Project Medishare/University of Miami; set up using Cirque de Soleil tents: Haiti Earthquake 2011.

quite a bit in disaster. This has proved to be more harmful than undertriage.[6] Triage tags provide useful in disaster settings (**Fig. 7**). Red means immediate and that the patient is critical and survival is likely if treatment is initiated early. Examples of this could include brain bleeds, tension pneumothorax, or intraabdominal bleeding. Yellow means urgent and the patient still can be critical; however, they are likely okay to wait a few hours before receiving treatment. This could include pelvic or spinal or compound fractures. Green means nonurgent and stable for hours up to several days.

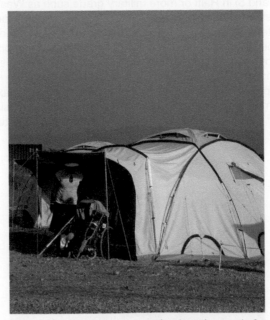

Fig. 5. Isolation tents: Haiti earthquake; predominately used for TB patients. TB, tuberculosis.

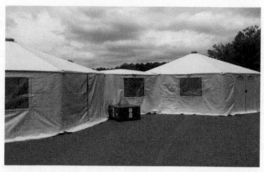

Fig. 6. Western shelter: DMAT field hospital: Center of Disaster Preparedness Training site.

Minor lacerations, sprains, and simple fractures could fall into this category. Placing a black tag on a patient means that this patient is likely to be dead soon. No medical care is likely to help this patient.[2,8,9]

Providers should remember the golden hour in trauma surgery which is the first 60 minutes following the trauma where patients have the highest likelihood of surviving if given prompt surgical treatment. This means we need to look and see where our patient might be bleeding. It could be into the head so a rapid neuro examination consisting of mental status examination and pupillary light response should be performed. Computed tomographic scans might not be readily available. The provider should next start to scan down the body, viewing any neck or vessel injuries, then to the chest thinking if there could be any possible hemo/pneumothorax or broken ribs. A chest radiograph can be performed if the site has set up for mobile imaging. If the provider has an ultrasound it is recommended that a pericardial and pleural ultrasound be performed. Bilateral chest tubes or needle aspiration may be indicated. Ultrasound may also be used for many parts of the body including neck, chest, and abdomen in a focused abdominal sonographic test for trauma (FAST examination).[10] Bedside diagnostic peritoneal aspiration is not frequently used anymore; however, on the field it may be useful to identify any blood in the abdomen quickly. The pelvis should be scanned for any perineal or scrotal hematomas and rocked for any instability. Extremities should be scanned

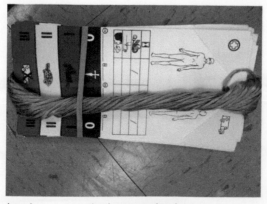

Fig. 7. Triage tags placed on or attached to people's bodies.

for hemorrhage or any compartment swelling, especially in the thigh, as it may indicate a broken femur that the patient will potentially bleed to death from. Other areas that should be surveyed include the scalp, back, and perineum. Providers should ask about blood pressure on the field if it was taken, as patients may have been hypotensive in the field and their body may be compensating on arrival and seem normal and be exsanguinating inside. Spinal cord injury should always be suspected. If the patient has unidentified shock, a laparotomy and pericardial window can be performed.[11] Makeshift operating rooms (ORs) can help with this.

MAKESHIFT OPERATING ROOMS

When setting up field hospitals more so than clinics, a tent or a section of a tent is set up to become a makeshift OR (**Fig. 8**). This may not even be a room. There may just be sterile blue curtains set up. The intensive care unit may be behind those curtains and OR supplies stored in the back (**Fig. 9**). There may be dust, dirt, and sand all over the floors. The operating theater may be the furthest from sterile. Those who arrive into your OR may be ones who might not need emergent surgical care, those who are in extremis, or those who need emergent surgery, which is why it is important to scan the person and perform a rapid assessment of the injured.[12]

There is what is known as damage control resuscitation and damage control surgery. Damage control resuscitation includes giving blood, coagulation, and fluids in attempts to stabilize the patient. Hemostatic dressings and tourniquets are sometimes included in the resuscitation terminology. Damage control surgery relates to trying to stop hypothermia, coagulopathy, and acidosis.[12] Initially, surgery is performed in attempts to stop the hemorrhage. Fluids and blood products are given to then attempt to stop the coagulopathy and acid base disorders occurring. Then when the patient is more stable they are returned to the OR to repair the injuries.[13]

Debridement and leaving wounds open after thoroughly irrigating and delaying closure have had the best outcomes on the field.[6]

PREPARING

There is not one way for a provider to prepare for a disaster. There are many helpful classes, including the Definitive Surgical Trauma Care (DSTC) Course, Advanced Surgical Skill Exposure in Trauma (ASSET), Emergency War Surgery (EWS), Tactical

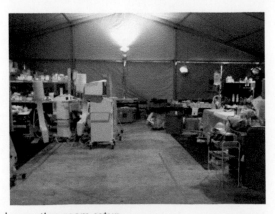

Fig. 8. Storage and operating room setup.

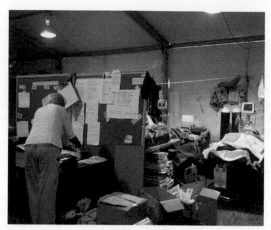

Fig. 9. Makeshift ICU in a tent: Haiti earthquake.

Combat Casualty Course (TCCC), The Trauma and Evaluation Management Team (TEAM), Aeromedical trainings, and the Intensive Care and the Damage Control Surgery courses organized by European Association of Trauma and Emergency Surgery.[7,14] Advanced trauma life support and prehospital trauma life support are also recommended. Participating in your institution's mass casualty incident (MCI) drills or joining a state run or medical reserve committee drill can greatly prepare providers for the field. Providers after the Boston bombing and Las Vegas shootings were well organized and had participated in many MCI drills.[15,16] There are also several other programs run by organizations such as The Red Cross, Humanitarian Learning Center, and FEMA trainings in the ICS system.

When working in disaster surgery, providers should learn how to use equipment they might see on the field, such as an ISTAT and Ultrasound to perform a focused abdominal ultrasound test for trauma (FAST). Combat Application Tourniquets (CAT) are recommended for providers going into disaster situations. CATs were assessed in 145 servicemen, and Doppler were used to see if blood flow was impeded. Only 70% of participants successfully cut off blood supply.[17] So, although having this in your tool kit is important, it is more important to learn how to properly use it. Providers should also remember their physical examination skills, as the basics are key to diagnosing in most situations unless your team has a supply cache.

When on the ground, providers should get to know their team. They should learn everyone's names or create name tags. Providers should also learn what resources are available to them and their team. [12,18]

In a disaster setting, one will not have their typical operating equipment. Surgical equipment may not be what one is used to, ventilators may be different to those you are accustomed to, syringes may be with different measurement units, overhead lighting might be resorted to a head-lamp, oxygen may not be readily available, and even temperature cannot be controlled for the environment or the patient.[19] In Haiti, Gigli saws were used for both amputations and then craniotomies.[20] Surgeons will not have their favorite scrub nurse or tech to work with. Physician assistants will have to work with many providers unknown to them and may have to perform procedures they typically might not do. Task and role sharing may be common in disaster settings. Familiarizing oneself with the makeshift OR is essential. One cannot rely on someone else to know where something is. Each individual should take responsibility in this. One should identify where your pediatric equipment is located because many times there is a shortage of supplies for children.[8] In remote and rural areas pediatric referral facilities may not be easily accessible.[11]

Disaster teams should also look to other organizations and communicate if needing help. In Haiti, there was a shortage of oxygen tanks, and the Israeli army was able to help supply oxygen for critical patients. In the Bahamas, a large pharmaceutical company that had a relationship with a disaster organization donated 1000 units of tetanus to one NGO, and this dire product was shared with many other organizations that needed it (**Fig. 10**).

STERILIZATION/PREOPERATIVE/OPERATIVE CARE

When it comes to WaSH and hand washing, running water is not always readily available. Hand scrub solutions such as chlorhexidine and alcohol-based gels can be used. In Haiti OR equipment was washed down with bleach, ortho-phthalaldehyde, and 2% hydrogen peroxide. A small steam autoclave arrived and was able to be used for sterilization. Glutaraldehyde solution 2% can also be used for sterilization of surfaces and instruments.[4]

Preoperatively, patients can be prepped with the above solutions with the exception of bleach. Preoperative antibiotics should be given if they are available. Tetanus toxoid and immune globin should also be administered. In Haiti, less than 50% percent of the population had been vaccinated.[20] I saw my first ever case of tetanus in Haiti.

Nothing by mouth (NPO) in disaster surgery is not always possible. Sometimes patients are so malnourished and dehydrated and supplies of crystalloids are limited that the provider may have to be liberal with their NPO policies before and after surgery.

Surgical Safety-Checklists such as those from the WHO (**Fig. 11**) should still be verified.[21] Providers should make sure they have the correct patient, the right site, adequate fluids, and informed consent and introduce themselves and their roles to the team. Consent is usually verbal in a disaster setting and can be obtained from the patient, family, or translators.

Communication with patients can be very difficult in this setting, as language and cultural barriers may be present. Some patients in Haiti expressed they rather be dead than have an amputation and refused surgeries despite multiple providers trying to educate them on the complications that may ensue.

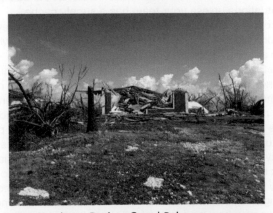

Fig. 10. Destruction post-Hurricane Dorian: Grand Bahama

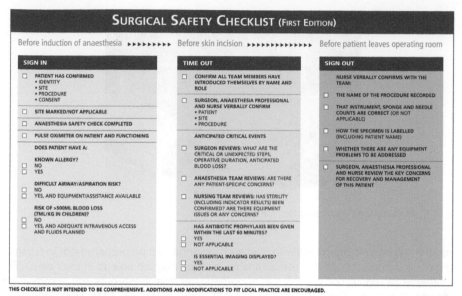

SURGICAL SAFETY CHECKLIST (First Edition)

Before induction of anaesthesia ►►►►►►►► Before skin incision ►►►►►►►►►►► Before patient leaves operating room

SIGN IN	TIME OUT	SIGN OUT
☐ PATIENT HAS CONFIRMED • IDENTITY • SITE • PROCEDURE • CONSENT	☐ CONFIRM ALL TEAM MEMBERS HAVE INTRODUCED THEMSELVES BY NAME AND ROLE	NURSE VERBALLY CONFIRMS WITH THE TEAM:
☐ SITE MARKED/NOT APPLICABLE	☐ SURGEON, ANAESTHESIA PROFESSIONAL AND NURSE VERBALLY CONFIRM • PATIENT • SITE • PROCEDURE	☐ THE NAME OF THE PROCEDURE RECORDED
☐ ANAESTHESIA SAFETY CHECK COMPLETED		☐ THAT INSTRUMENT, SPONGE AND NEEDLE COUNTS ARE CORRECT (OR NOT APPLICABLE)
☐ PULSE OXIMETER ON PATIENT AND FUNCTIONING	ANTICIPATED CRITICAL EVENTS	☐ HOW THE SPECIMEN IS LABELLED (INCLUDING PATIENT NAME)
DOES PATIENT HAVE A:	☐ SURGEON REVIEWS: WHAT ARE THE CRITICAL OR UNEXPECTED STEPS, OPERATIVE DURATION, ANTICIPATED BLOOD LOSS?	☐ WHETHER THERE ARE ANY EQUIPMENT PROBLEMS TO BE ADDRESSED
KNOWN ALLERGY? ☐ NO ☐ YES	☐ ANAESTHESIA TEAM REVIEWS: ARE THERE ANY PATIENT-SPECIFIC CONCERNS?	☐ SURGEON, ANAESTHESIA PROFESSIONAL AND NURSE REVIEW THE KEY CONCERNS FOR RECOVERY AND MANAGEMENT OF THIS PATIENT
DIFFICULT AIRWAY/ASPIRATION RISK? ☐ NO ☐ YES, AND EQUIPMENT/ASSISTANCE AVAILABLE	☐ NURSING TEAM REVIEWS: HAS STERILITY (INCLUDING INDICATOR RESULTS) BEEN CONFIRMED? ARE THERE EQUIPMENT ISSUES OR ANY CONCERNS?	
RISK OF >500ML BLOOD LOSS (7ML/KG IN CHILDREN)? ☐ NO ☐ YES, AND ADEQUATE INTRAVENOUS ACCESS AND FLUIDS PLANNED	HAS ANTIBIOTIC PROPHYLAXIS BEEN GIVEN WITHIN THE LAST 60 MINUTES? ☐ YES ☐ NOT APPLICABLE	
	IS ESSENTIAL IMAGING DISPLAYED? ☐ YES ☐ NOT APPLICABLE	

THIS CHECKLIST IS NOT INTENDED TO BE COMPREHENSIVE. ADDITIONS AND MODIFICATIONS TO FIT LOCAL PRACTICE ARE ENCOURAGED.

Fig. 11. WHO safety checklist. (*From* https://www.who.int/teams/integrated-health-services/patient-safety/research/safe-surgery.)

Depending on the environment, general anesthesia is not always used if access to electricity, generators, or ventilators is not stable. Ketamine was used in Haiti quite frequently for conscious sedation.[20] Anesthesiologists and nurse anesthetists might not always be available, and surgeons and providers might have to control their own procedures.

In Haiti operating tables were made of wood planks and covered with blue sterile drapes. The Bahamas had flood waters surge their ORs, and it was several days before a surgical field hospital was set up by Good Samaritan's Purse (**Fig. 12**). The

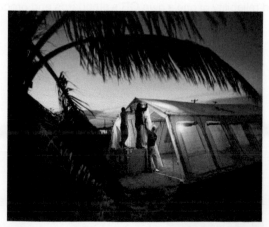

Fig. 12. Field hospital setup. Photo by Good Samaritan's Purse; Grand Bahama post-Hurricane Dorian.

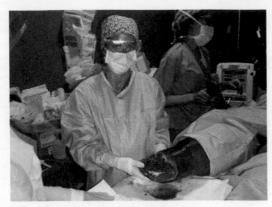

Fig. 13. Amputations common after Haiti earthquake.

provider will have to improvise with their surroundings and be prepared not to finish a surgery to completion as they would like to, as they may be able to in their own OR.

External fixations, not closing the abdomen, multiple wash-outs are common in disaster surgeries (**Fig. 13**). Infections are very common after limb injuries[17] (**Fig. 14**). Postsurgical infections and complications are rampant after a disaster. The conditions are far from sterile. Providers need to be diligent in checking wounds, providing proper wound care instructions and supplies to patients. Patients will not be able to obtain their own supplies, as many stores and pharmacies will have been destroyed. Patients should have follow-up plans detailed out and ensure that some setup is in place for other providers to know what the patient's situation was. Many providers come and go into disaster zones, as staying in them for very long periods of time can be very stressful. Providers should be prepared to be working with multiple different people, limited resources, and having limited reports on their patients.

TEAMWORK

Disasters are times of high stress. Not everyone will feel comfortable in austere environments. Water, showering, personal habits, and space will be lost.[22] The comforts of the knowledge and reliability of one's own OR's standards and procedures will not be

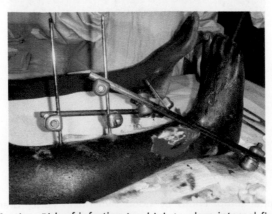

Fig. 14. External fixation. Risk of infection too high to place internal fixation.

present. Team members may become easily frustrated or one will notice a sense of desperation or exhaustion. Signs to watch out that your teammate is becoming traumatized are that they are becoming more and more cynical, they may seem distant, they isolate themselves, or they begin speaking very negatively. Providers need to encourage each other in these environments. It is a conscious effort to ensure that your teammates are ok.

DOCUMENTATION/COMMUNICATION

After a disaster, electronic medical records are usually inaccessible. After the 2010 earthquake in Haiti, patient names were not easily accessible, and there was a need to individually collect each name to create a database for family and other survivors to find each other.[23] Many patients at that time did not even had photo or government identification with them. Personal Health information should still be maintained. Providers should remember not to take pictures of patients. In areas where cell phones are not working, 2-way radios cannot be guaranteed to be encrypted so coded terminology should be used.[14] Paper documentation can be clipped to the bedside; however, at times this gets lost too. Typically, notes have been written on the patient's bandages to include date, surgery performed, packed red blood cells transfused, and next anticipated procedure, as well as if any packs were left inside the patient.

With the multiple federal, state, tribal, and NGO teams on the ground, communication is lacking. Meetings with PAHO/WHO have stressed for the need for international standards and greater accountability in order to have improved data and knowledge of the situation on the ground.[5] It is essential after a disaster to collect this information. Templates have been created from institutions such as Medecins Sans Frontieres and other NGOs, but not everyone is aware of reporting back to the proper authorities. As a provider at a surgical site, one should ensure that they are documenting and delivering the information to the appropriate entities. This information is essential for national authorities and the WHO's Global Health Cluster to reduce morbidity, mortality, decrease public health emergencies, follow epidemics, ensure equipment and supplies get to areas, and reduce duplication of efforts. This will also allow for the following of patient care and those that are moved from their home community to receive advanced care.

EVACUATION

In Nepal, after the 2015 earthquake, 2 patients were evacuated via helicopter from a mission in the Ganesh Mountain region. These patients needed surgical care, and a field hospital was not able to perform these procedures. This required the team to find appropriate landing zones, mark out the perimeters for the landing site, and assess wind conditions and shift positions rapidly if need be, as well as stay in constant communication with the pilots. The patients would not make the 4-day walk to Kathmandu, so evacuation was the only way to ensure a mother with eclampsia safely delivered her baby and a man who was running and fell onto a stick that lodged into his sinuses would not become septic. The team communicated the evacuations with authorities and the WHO.

In disasters such as Haiti and the Bahamas field hospitals were able to provide surgical care; however, some patients still needed to be evacuated for higher level of care. Working with Project Medishare, a University of Miami Hospital that had strong ties in Haiti before the earthquake, teams are able to transport patients to the USS Comfort, and many patients were transported via private planes to accepting surgeons in university hospitals along the Florida coast. Many critical patients were evacuated initially by US Coast Guard off the Abacos Islands and Grand Bahama to Nassau. Not knowing the patient's identity, minimal documentation, and limited space on aircrafts, patients were oftentimes separated from their families.

FAMILY

When family could be identified, they played a huge role with assisting providers. They could tell us a patient's name and their medical history, occasionally act as translators, help carry patients, do wound care once trained by us, and once discharged help ensure that the patient was able to return to us for follow-up care. Patient families even helped with waste removal in Haiti.[20] It was very difficult when families are not identified, as when transferring patients to the United States from Haiti, and little information was known about the patient. In Haiti teams were allowed to transport people with emergency VISAs to the United States; however, that did not mean the family was always allowed to come along with the patient. This strained communication with family and on return to country of origin, follow-up care became increasingly difficult.

FOLLOW-UP CARE

On a good day with normal conditions, patients who have surgery get lost to follow-up care. Patients may not show backup for a post-op visit due to several reasons such as cost, transport, logistics, and/or feeling that they are fine. In a disaster setting, this all can become much more confusing, as the patient may not have a home anymore and may be living in a makeshift tent, they may not have a car, or they may not have any of the valid documentation to prove who they are to access their financial accounts. Many different providers have typically rotated in and out to see the patient; documentation is scarce and patients are not always sure of what procedure they have had done. For this reason, complications and postsurgical infections are common after disaster. Many external fixations were placed after the 2010 Haiti earthquake and many remained on many months after, as patients did not know where to return or understand what to do with them.

SUMMARY

Understanding key concepts for disaster surgery is not just a military phenomenon. Providers can be faced with a disaster and sparse working conditions at any moment from a natural to a man-made disaster. The goal is to perform damage control surgery, stabilize the patient, and transfer the patient to a tertiary center or provide detailed follow-up for the patient. Providers need to learn who they are working with and keep up their skills sets. Working with limited resources and the possible inability to transfer patients out may create high levels of stress and fatigue. Continuing to check on one's team is an important dynamic to working in disaster surgery. Working in disaster takes dedication, teamwork, cultural competency, and perseverance.

CLINICS CARE POINTS

- Pearls: participate in disaster drills and trainings prior to a disaster Learn how to use the field equipment ASAP; ask for help if you do not know as you may be the one responsible for it at any given time Ensure you know where equipment is located and stored in a field hospital.

- Pitfalls: Not introducing yourself to your team and understanding everyone's roles/responsibilities Assuming someone else will get the job done; everyone in disaster is plays a role in task-sharing Expecting certain supplies; providers must work with what is available.

DISCLOSURE

The views/opinions expressed are those of the authors and do not necessarily represent the views of the Yale School of Medicine. No other relevant disclosures or conflicts of interest exist.

REFERENCES

1. Joshua St. Clair. Pararescue - The special ops unit that rescues Navy SEALS. Esquire. 2019. Available at: https://www.esquire.com/news-politics/a28692306/us-air-force-pararescue-tamar-rescue-mission/. Accessed January 6, 2020.
2. Mamoon Rashid. Disaster Surgery. In: Williams N, O'Connell PR, editors. Bailey & Love's Short Practice of Surgery; 2018:409-423.
3. Unit 3 disaster sequence of events. Available at: https://training.fema.gov/emiweb/downloads/is208sdmunit3.pdf. Accessed August 15, 2019.
4. Briggs SM. Disaster preparedness and response. In: surgery during natural disasters, combat, terrorist attacks, and crisis situations. Cham (Switzerland): Springer International Publishing; 2016. p. 7–18.
5. Burkle FM, Nickerson JW, von Schreeb J, et al. Emergency surgery data and documentation reporting forms for sudden-onset humanitarian crises, natural disasters and the existing burden of surgical disease. Prehospital Disaster Med 2012. https://doi.org/10.1017/S1049023X12001306.
6. Jamkar A, Jamkar A, Roy N, et al. The leadership role of surgeons in disaster management. Indian J Surg 2013;75(4):253–4.
7. Lennquist S, Lennquist S. Education and training in disaster medicine do we need to train our surgeons for disasters? Vol 94. 2005. Available at: https://journals.sagepub.com/doi/pdf/10.1177/145749690509400409. Accessed June 5, 2019.
8. Showstark M, Lovejoy B. Crisis standards of care. Physician Assist Clin 2019; 4(4):663–73.
9. Dicker RA, Adams JE. The experience of disaster response in Sri Lanka: from reaction to planning the future. In: surgery during natural disasters, combat, terrorist attacks, and crisis situations. Cham (Switzerland): Springer International Publishing; 2016. p. 103–12.
10. Choi YU. Awake tracheostomy in an austere setting. In: surgery during natural disasters, combat, terrorist attacks, and crisis situations. Cham (Switzerland): Springer International Publishing; 2016. p. 73–6.
11. Martin MJ, Yach ZMS, Eckert MJ. Pediatric emergencies in the combat or austere environment: as easy as A, B, C! In: surgery during natural disasters, combat, terrorist attacks, and crisis situations. Cham (Switzerland): Springer International Publishing; 2016. p. 77–95.
12. Lim CRB, editor. Surgery during natural disasters, combat, terrorist attacks, and crisis situations. Cham (Switzerland): Springer International Publishing; 2016.
13. Black GE, Steele SR. Surgery under fire. In: surgery during natural disasters, combat, terrorist attacks, and crisis situations. Cham (Switzerland): Springer International Publishing; 2016. p. 165–79.

14. Jones S, Wisbach G. Trauma surgery in an austere environment: trauma and emergency surgery in unusual situations. In: surgery during natural disasters, combat, terrorist attacks, and crisis situations. Cham (Switzerland): Springer International Publishing; 2016. p. 19–45.

15. Shultz JM, Thoresen S, Galea S. The las vegas shootings—underscoring key features of the firearm epidemic. JAMA 2017;318(18):1753.

16. King DR, Mesar T. Lessons learned from the boston marathon bombing. In: surgery during natural disasters, combat, terrorist attacks, and crisis situations. Cham (Switzerland): Springer International Publishing; 2016. p. 181–90.

17. Ashkenazi I, Bemelman M. Editorial: "focus on disaster and military surgery. Eur J Trauma Emerg Surg 2017;43(5):575–7.

18. Lim CRB. Operating in a tent. In: surgery during natural disasters, combat, terrorist attacks, and crisis situations. Cham (Switzerland): Springer International Publishing; 2016. p. 139–48.

19. Bulger EM, Briggs SM. A surgical response to the Haiti earthquake 2010. In: surgery during natural disasters, combat, terrorist attacks, and crisis situations. Cham (Switzerland): Springer International Publishing; 2016. p. 113–23.

20. Jawa RS, Zakrison TL, Richards AT, et al. Facilitating safer surgery and anesthesia in a disaster zone. Am J Surg 2012;204(3):406–9.

21. World Health Organization. WHO Surgical Safety Checklist. (First Edition). Availble at: https://www.who.int/teams/integrated-health-services/patient-safety/research/safe-surgery/tool-and-resources.

22. Showstark M. Serving the Underserved Internationally. Physician Assist Clin 2019;4(1):xxi–xxxix.

23. Post-earthquake injuries treated at a field hospital — Haiti,. 2010. Available at: https://www.cdc.gov/mmwr/preview/mmwrhtml/mm5951a1.htm. Accessed October 8, 2019.

Surgical Wound Infections

Carey L. Barry, MHS, PA-C, MT(ASCP)

KEYWORDS

- Surgical site infection (SSI) • Surgical wound infection • Surgical prophylaxis
- Hospital acquired infection (HAI)

KEY POINTS

- Surgical site infections are among the most common hospital-acquired infections in the United States.
- Surgical site infections are classified by extent of involvement: superficial incisional, deep incisional, and organ/space surgical site infections.
- Guidelines for prevention of surgical site infections include parental antimicrobial prophylaxis, alcohol-based skin preparation, perioperative glycemic control, and maintenance of normothermia.

INTRODUCTION

The work of Louis Pasteur, Joseph Lister, and Robert Koch in the late nineteenth century has informed the role of infection on surgical outcomes and ultimately served as the foundation for the transformation of surgical medicine.

Louis Pasteur was a French scientist whose studies in fermentation, anthrax, silkworm disease, chicken cholera, and rabies led to the development of the germ theory of fermentation and subsequently the germ theory of disease.[1-3] In his early fermentation studies, he proposed that microorganisms caused fermentation and decomposition during a time when it was widely believed to be solely a chemical reaction. He developed techniques of sterilizing equipment in the laboratory that later would translate into similar applications in the surgical setting.

British surgeon Joseph Lister brought his experience and observations as a surgeon and his belief in the germ theory of disease to his development of aseptic techniques using carbolic acid in the surgical setting.[4] He developed a set of principles in asepsis to be used in approach to surgery and surgical wounds: (1) destroy germs on the patient's skin, the surgeon's hands, the instruments, and the area surrounding the surgical site; (2) prevent germs from the air from entering the wound during surgery; and (3) prevent germs from entering the wound after surgery.[3-6]

Physician Assistant Program, Bouvé College of Health Sciences, Northeastern University, 202 Robinson Hall, 360 Huntington Avenue, Boston, MA 02115, USA
E-mail address: c.barry@northeastern.edu

Physician Assist Clin 6 (2021) 295–307
https://doi.org/10.1016/j.cpha.2020.11.003
2405-7991/21/© 2020 The Author. Published by Elsevier Inc.
physicianassistant.theclinics.com

Robert Koch was a German physician who had experience with wound infections during his service at a battlefield hospital. His research working with anthrax and his discovery of *Mycobacterium tuberculosis* would serve as a foundation for what came to be known as Koch postulates. These postulates would establish a causal relationship between a specific microorganism and disease.[3,7]

In the era prior to these discoveries and the development and implementation of the principles of asepsis, infection after surgery was an expected outcome. Purulence that was localized to the surgical wound was considered a favorable outcome. A local infection could be treated successfully, but a widespread infection likely would be fatal. Morbidity and mortality due to surgical wound infections decreased with the implementation of surgical asepsis. These discoveries and innovations of the late nineteenth century marked the beginning of the evolution of surgical care and remain at the core of knowledge of surgical site infections (SSIs).[1–3]

DEFINITION AND CLASSIFICATION
Surgical Site Infection

A surgical wound infection involves an infection at the surgical incision site after an operation. Use of the term, surgical wound infection, has been modified to SSI, to better represent infections at the surgical site and not just the incision.[8] The Centers for Disease Control and Prevention (CDC) define SSI as any infection after surgery the involves the surgical wound (incision) or organ/space that was manipulated during the procedure that occurs within 30 days of surgery or within 1 year with prosthetic material implantation. SSIs are classified as superficial incisional SSI, deep incisional SSI, or organ/space SSI (see **Table 1** for criteria).[8] A suture abscess or stitch abscess is an abscess at the suture site only and is not considered an SSI. Remote infections resulting from surgery but not involving the surgical site are called surgical patient infections.[8] An example of a surgical patient infection is pneumonia or a urinary tract infection in a patient who underwent an appendectomy.

ETIOLOGY

Surgical manipulation of tissue causes changes in host (patient) defense mechanisms against infection. Skin and mucous membranes provide a physical barrier to pathogens and bacteria entering a patient's tissues.[2] Additionally, the skin and mucous membranes of normal healthy individuals are colonized with bacteria collectively known as normal microbial flora. Normal microbial flora varies slightly between individual people, but there are common types of bacteria found in specific anatomic locations (**Table 2**).[9–11] Disruption of this barrier during surgical procedures can allow normal microbial flora and other pathogens to enter the surrounding tissues, which can lead to infection. Further manipulation of tissue or organs in the surgical site during the operation can expose the surgical site to bacterial flora typically present at the specific site. Introduction of bacteria can occur from external sources of contamination during the procedure or after the procedure. Exposure to microorganisms stimulates an immune response in the patient. If the microbes are not eliminated by a patient's immune response, an infection develops. The resulting infection can be contained, locoregional, or systemic[2] (**Box 1**). Although most SSIs are bacterial, infections can be fungal or viral in origin.[2] Common bacterial pathogens involved in SSIs are listed in **Table 3**. The most common bacterial pathogens involved are *Staphylococcus aureus* (methicillin-resistant *Staphylococcus aureus* [MRSA] and methicillin-sensitive *Staphylococcus aureus* [MSSA]), coagulase-negative staphylococci, and enterococci.[12,13]

Table 1
Surgical site infections are classified into 3 categories: superficial incisional, deep incisional (fascia and muscle), and organ/space criteria for surgical site infection[8]

Surgical Site Infection General Criteria	Classification	Structures	Criteria
• Infection related to an operative procedure • Occurs at or near surgical site • Within 30 d of procedure[b]	Superficial incisional SSI	Skin Subcutaneous tissue	General criteria AND 1 of the following: • Purulent drainage from superficial incision (not deep) • Organisms isolated from aseptically obtained culture • ≥1 sign or symptom pain/tenderness, localized swelling, erythema, warmth, or superficial incision deliberately opened (unless culture is negative)
	Deep incisional SSI	Deep soft tissue (fascia and muscle)	General criteria AND 1 of the following: • Purulent drainage from deep incision (not organ space) • Spontaneous dehisces or deliberately opened with fever and/or pain/tenderness (unless culture is negative) • Abscess or evidence of infection on direct examination, during reoperation, or by histologic or radiologic examination
	Organ/space SSI	Organ/space	General criteria and involves any part of the anatomy (organ or space) opened or manipulated during the procedure (specific sites assigned to identify location[a]) AND 1 of the following: • Purulent drainage from a drain placed through stab wound into the organ/space • Organisms isolated from aseptically obtained culture of fluid or tissue • Abscess or evidence of infection involving organ/space on direct on direct examination, during reoperation, or by histologic or radiologic examination

[a] Specific sites of organ/space SSI: arterial or venous infection, breast abscess or mastitis, disc space, ear/mastoid, endometritis, endocarditis, eye (not conjunctivitis), gastrointestinal tract, intra-abdominal, intracranial, brain, dural infections abscesses, joint or bursa, mediastinitis, meningitis or ventriculitis, myocarditis or pericarditis, oral cavity (mouth, tongue, or gums), osteomyelitis, other lower respiratory tract infection, other urinary tract infections, other male or female reproductive tract, spinal abscess without meningitis, sinusitis, upper respiratory tract, pharyngitis, and vaginal cuff (episiotomy, circumcision, and burn wounds are excluded).
[b] Within 1 y if prosthetic material is implanted and seems associated with operative site for deep incisional or organ/space SSI.

Table 2
Normal microbial flora: the normal microbial flora commonly is called microbiota

| Anatomic Location | Gram Positive | | Gram Negative | |
	Cocci	Rods	Cocci	Rods
Skin	Staphylococcus epidermidis Staphylococcus aureus Micrococcus α-Hemolytic streptococci Nonhemolytic streptococci Peptostreptococcus species Propionibacterium species	Corynebacterium species Propionibacterium acnes		Enteric bacilli (some sites) Acinetobacter species (coccobacilli)
Nasopharynx	α-Hemolytic streptococci Staphylococcus epidermidis Nonhemolytic streptococci Micrococcus Anaerobes	Corynebacterium	Neisseria species (nonpathogenic)	Haemophilus species Prevotella species Anaerobes
Gastrointestinal tract (stomach) Small flora* (undetectable to 10^3/g of contents)	*Limited to bacteria swallowed with food	Lactobacillus species		
Gastrointestinal tract (ileum) Moderate mixed flora (10^6/g to 10^8/g of contents)	Enterococci			Enterobacteriaceae
Gastrointestinal tract (large intestine) Dense flora (10^9/g to 10^{11}/g of contents)	Streptococcus Enterococci α-Hemolytic streptococci non-hemolytic streptococci Anaerobes Peptostreptococcus species	Lactobacillus species Clostridium species Diphtheroids		Enterobacteriaceae Bacteroides Enteric bacilli Anaerobes
Genitalia	Streptococcus α-Hemolytic streptococci Nonhemolytic streptococci	Lactobacillus species Corynebacterium species	Neisseria species (nonpathogenic)	Bacteroides Anaerobes

This is a small representation of some of the most common bacteria in the microbiota of specific anatomic locations.[9–11]
* the Small flora is limited to the bacteria swallowed with food.

Box 1
Degree of infection

Contained infection
- Local purulence
- Furuncle
- Abscess

Locoregional with or without distant spread
- Cellulitis
- Lymphangitis
- Aggressive soft tissue infection
- Metastatic abscess

Systemic infection
- Bacteremia
- Fungemia
- Systemic inflammatory response syndrome
- Sepsis
- Septic shock

RISK FACTORS

There are many risk factors for developing an SSI, including microbe-related factors, patient factors, and procedure-related factors (**Box 2**).[2,15–20] Degree of wound contamination has been shown to be a risk factor for development of SSI; a classification of wound by degree of contamination is found in **Table 4**.[21–23]

IMPACT AND PREVENTATIVE MEASURES

SSIs remain a significant burden, with approximately 2% to 5% of patients undergoing inpatient surgery developing an SSI.[2,14,26,27] Although there has been a decrease in the prevalence of SSIs, SSIs remain among the most common hospital-acquired infections (HAIs) in the United States, representing approximately 21.8% of all HAIs.[26,28–30] SSIs remain a significant burden, resulting in increased morbidity and mortality, extended postoperative recovery, increased use of health care resources, and cost of approximately $20,785 per case in the United States.[27,31,32]

The importance of prevention of SSIs is reflected in the ongoing research and the updated guidelines by 4 major organizations over the past several years: the World Health Organization (WHO), CDC, American College of Surgeons (ACS), and Surgical Infection Society (SIS).[32–34] **Table 5** summarizes the strongest recommendations across recently published guidelines and literature.[32–35].

There are many other studies evaluating preventative measures and risk assessment for developing an SSI with interesting findings and varying support for implementation. Recent studies have shown no reduction in SSI with the use of disposable surgical jackets or the use of a bouffant head covers over allowing a choice in surgical head-wear while in the operating room.[37,38] The use of negative pressure dressings had mixed results in studies with no consistent benefit demonstrated.[39–41] Decolonization of patients who are carriers of *Staphylococcus aureus* prior to surgery has been recommended in the ACS and SIS guidelines and by the WHO guidelines, and there is evidence that this could reduce SSIs.[42–44] ERAS or bundling of perioperative care has gained interest and has had promising results in specific fields but needs further development and investigation prior to widespread adoption.[45–47]

Table 3
Common bacterial surgical pathogens: most surgical site infections are bacterial[2,14]

	Gram Positive		Gram Negative	
	Cocci	Rods	Cocci	Rods
Aerobic	Staphylococcus aureus			Escherichia coli
	Coagulase-negative staphylococci			Haemophilus influenzae (coccobacilli)
	Staphylococcus epidermidis			Klebsiella pneumoniae
	Streptococcus pyogenes			Proteus mirabilis
	Streptococcus pneumoniae			Enterobacter cloacae
	Enterococcus faecium			Enterobacter aerogenes
	Enterococcus faecalis			Serratia marcescens
				Acinetobacter calcoacetisus (coccobacilli)
				Citrobacter freundii
				Pseudomonas aeruginosa
				Stenotrophomonas maltophilia
Anaerobes	Peptostreptococcus species	Clostridium difficile		Bacteroides fragilis
		Clostridium perfringens		Fusobacterium species
		Clostridium tetani		
		Clostridium septicum		
Other	Mycobacterium avium-intracellulare			
	Mycobacterium tuberculosis			
	Nocardia asteroids			
	Legionella pneumophilia			
	Listeria monocytogenes			

Box 2
The risk factors for surgical site infection (SSI) fall in three categories[2,15,17,19,20,24,25]

MICROBE RELATED
- Degree of wound contamination
- Virulence of pathogen
- Prolonged hospitalization prior to surgery

PATIENT RELATED
- Index of disease
- Morbid obesity
- Advanced age
- Protein-calorie malnutrition
- Age
- Immunosuppressants
- Diabetes mellitus
- Smoking
- Cancer
- Systemic infection

OPERATION RELATED
- Duration of operation (>2 hours)
- Tissue trauma
- Poor hemostasis
- Presence of foreign material
- Intra-abdominal procedure
- Technique

Table 4
Wound classification according to degree of contamination[21]

Contamination Classification	Definition[a]	Surgical Site Infection Rates[21]
Clean	These are uninfected operative wounds in which no inflammation is encountered and the respiratory, alimentary, genital, or uninfected urinary tracts are not entered.	1.76% Superficial incisional 0.54% Deep incisional 0.28% Organ/space
Clean/contaminated	These are operative wounds in which the respiratory, alimentary, genital, or urinary tract is entered under controlled conditions and without unusual contamination.	3.94% Superficial incisional 0.86% Deep incisional 1.87% Organ/space
Contaminated	These include open, fresh, accidental wounds; operations with major breaks in sterile technique or gross spillage from the gastrointestinal tract; and incisions in which acute, nonpurulent inflammation is encountered.	4.75% Superficial incisional 1.31% Deep incisional 2.55% Organ/space
Dirty	These include old traumatic wounds with retained devitalized tissue and those that involve existing clinical infection or perforated viscera.	5.16% Superficial incisional 2.1% Deep incisional 4.54% Organ/apace

[a] Classifications as defined by ACS National Surgical Quality Improvement Program.[21]

Table 5
Surgical site infection prophylaxis[32–35]

Recommendation	Summary of Guidelines
Parenteral antimicrobial prophylaxis	• Prior to skin incision • Antibiotics should be given so bactericidal concentration of agent is present during incision. • Antibiotics should be given within 60 min of incision, with redosing based on half-life of the antibiotic. • Discontinuation after skin closure in low-risk patients
Alcohol-based skin preparation[36]	• Alcohol-based preparations should be used unless contraindicated.
Perioperative glycemic control	• Target glucose levels <200 mg/dL versus 110–150 mg/dL • Preoperative and intraoperative warming
Temperature regulation to normothermia	• Perioperative normothermia is recommended. • Preoperative and intraoperative warming
Maintenance of normal tissue oxygen	• CDC: unclear indications • ACS/SIS and WHO: 80% supplemental oxygen preoperatively and possibly intraoperatively

CLINICAL PRESENTATION AND EVALUATION

SSI is a clinical diagnosis based on history and physical examination findings and can be confirmed with cultures. Criteria for diagnosis and classification of superficial incisional, deep incisional, and organ/space infections can be found in **Table 1**.[8] Routine assessment of surgical incisions begins shortly after surgery during the initial postoperative evaluation, then daily thereafter while in the hospital. In cases where the surgical dressing remains intact for several days after surgery, the surgical site is evaluated as best as possible through and around the dressing. Findings that are concerning for an SSI include pain or tenderness, erythema, warmth, induration, fluctuance, and purulent drainage at the surgical site. Fever, chills, tachycardia, tachypnea, and general feeling of illness are systemic signs and symptoms that are concerning for infection (**Box 3**). Erythema around staples or sutures can be due to a reaction to the foreign material and should not be confused with an SSI. Patients need to continue to monitor for signs and symptoms of infection once they return home postoperatively. Clear patient education should be provided with explicit instructions to notify the surgical provider if signs or symptoms of infection develop. If SSI is not clearly identifiable based on history and physical examination findings, the patient can be evaluated further with serial examinations for worsening signs or symptoms, imaging, or laboratory studies. The use of photography in remote postoperative assessment likely has some value but needs further investigation. One study showed the use of photography increased specificity in diagnosis of SSI but decreased sensitivity.[48]

Diagnostic studies are not always indicated but may include laboratory studies and diagnostic imaging based on a patient's clinical presentation. A complete blood cell count may show leukocytosis with increased neutrophils. Inflammatory markers, such as a C-reactive protein, may be useful for monitoring and diagnosis of osteomyelitis, but inflammatory markers can be elevated after surgery and should be

> **Box 3**
> **Surgical site infection: signs and symptoms**
>
> Local signs and symptoms
> - Pain or tenderness
> - Erythema
> - Warmth of the surgical site
> - Swelling
> - Induration
> - Drainage
> - Fluctuance or fluid collection
> - Wound separation/dehiscence
>
> Systemic signs and symptoms
> - Fever or sense of fever
> - Chills
> - Tachycardia
> - Tachypnea

interpreted in clinical context. A basic metabolic panel or comprehensive metabolic panel and coagulation studies may be indicated to evaluate organ function if systemic infection is suspected. Blood cultures should be obtained for persistent or recurrent fever or clinical suspicion for bacteremia. A Gram stain of the surgical site can be completed to guide early antibiotic selection beyond empiric therapy while awaiting cultures. Wound culture specimens need to be collected aseptically by cleansing the wound with saline and removing purulence and debris prior to collecting the specimen. Ideally, specimens for culture should be collected prior to initiation of antibiotic therapy, but treatment should not be delayed for specimen collection. A swab of the incision site commonly is collected, but tissue or fluid collection from suspected organ or space infections is preferred.[12] In addition to aerobic cultures, anaerobic, fungal, and mycobacterial cultures need to be considered at the time of reoperation in all organ/space infections and based on clinical suspicion or failure to improve for any SSI. Imaging studies can be utilized to assess for signs of infection, abscess, or extent of infection. Ultrasound, computed tomography, or magnetic resonance imaging can identify abscesses, fluid collections, or extent of infection, depending on the surgical site anatomic location. Systemic infections, sepsis, and septic shock are life-threatening conditions that could develop as a result of surgical infections; these conditions need to be addressed quickly and treated accordingly.

TREATMENT

The treatment of an SSI depends on multiple factors, including the extent of infection, tissue involved, the associated procedure, diagnostic and culture data, and presence of prosthetic material.

The principle goal of treating an SSI is to drain all purulence and débridement of devitalized or necrotic tissue.[2,14] If cellulitis alone is suspected near the surgical site, a trial of antibiotic therapy may be considered with close monitoring. If there is no improvement or there is worsening after a trial of antibiotic therapy, the incision must be opened, irrigated, and drained with débridement of any devitalized tissue. Superficial incisional infections can be treated with skin suture removal, drainage of purulence, irrigation, and débridement of any devitalized tissue. Antibiotics are indicated only in the following cases[2,14]:

> **Box 4**
> **The Infectious Diseases Society of America antibiotic recommendations[14]**
>
> - First-generation cephalosporin or antistaphylococcal penicillin for MSSA
> - Vancomycin or Linezolid or Daptomycin or Telavancin or Ceftaroline if at risk for MRSA (nasal colonization, history of MRSA, recent hospitalization, or recent antibiotics)
> - Agents against gram-negative bacteria and anaerobes such as cephalosporin PLUS metronidazole or fluoroquinolone PLUS metronidazole if at risk for gram-negative infection (surgery of the axilla, gastrointestinal tract, perineum, or female genital tract)

- Cellulitis (>5 cm from wound edge)
- Fever (>38.5°C)
- Tachycardia (>110 beats per minute)
- Leukocytosis (>12,000/µL)
- SSI plus systemic signs of infection in clean procedure on the trunk, head, neck, or extremities

Empiric antibiotic or antimicrobial selection is based on the initial Gram stain and the most likely pathogen or pathogens, taking into consideration the surgical site normal microbial flora (see **Table 2**), underlying disease process, known contamination at the time of the initial surgery, and common pathogens (**Box 4**, see **Table 3**).[2,14] Further antibiotic therapy should be guided by culture data and clinical course.[2,14] Patients who fail to improve need reevaluation for uncontrolled infection.

Aggressive soft tissue infections or necrotizing soft tissue infections require early and frequent débridement. Patients with organ/space or deep incisional SSIs may require débridement and/or washout of the organ or space involved in addition to antibiotic therapy. If prosthetic material is infected, removal typically is indicated. Ongoing local wound care may be needed to promote wound and incision healing.

SUMMARY

Great strides have been made since the discoveries and developments of Louis Pasteur, Joseph Lister, and Robert Koch. Surgical asepsis remains a fundamental aspect of surgical care today. Although the risk of surgical wound infection has decreased dramatically since the late nineteenth century, SSIs are among the most common HAIs. Further investigation in surgical prophylaxis and preventative measures are essential to continue to reduce the risk of surgical site infections.

CLINICS CARE POINTS

- Surgical site infection prophylaxis includes perioperative parental antimicrobial therapy, alcohol-based skin preparation, perioperative glycemic control, and maintenance of normothermia.
- Surgical site infection (SSI) is a clinical diagnosis based on history and physical examination findings.
- Signs and symptoms concerning for SSI can include surgical site tenderness or warmth, erythema, local swelling, induration, purulent drainage, fluid collection, wound separation/dehiscence, fever, chills, tachycardia, or tachypnea.
- Erythema around staples or sutures can be due to a reaction to the foreign material and should not be confused with an SSI.

- The principle goal of treating an SSI is to drain all purulence and debridement of devitalized or necrotic tissue.
- Antibiotics are indication only if there is cellulitis (>5 cm from wound edge), fever (>38.5°C), tachycardia (>110 beats per minute), leukocytosis (>12,000/mL), or SSI plus systemic signs of infection.
- Specimens for culture should be collected prior to initiation of antibiotic therapy, but treatment should not be delayed for specimen collection.

DISCLOSURE

The author has no disclosures. The author has no relationship with a commercial company that has a direct financial interest in subject matter or materials discussed in article or with a company making a competing product.

REFERENCES

1. Toledo-Pereyra LH. Louis pasteur surgical revolution. J Invest Surg 2009; 22(2):82–7.
2. Bulander RE, Dunn DL, Beilman GJ. Surgical infections. In: Brunicardi FC, Andersen DK, Billiar TR, et al, editors. Schwartz's principles of surgery, 11e. New York (NY): McGraw-Hill Education; 2019.
3. Gaynes RP. Germ theory medical pioneers in infectious diseases. In. Washington, DC. Washington, DC: ASM Press; 2011.
4. Lister J. Antiseptic principle of the practice of surgery. Hoboken (NJ): Generic NL Freebook Publisher; 1867.
5. Pitt D, Aubin J-M. Joseph Lister: Father Of Modern Surgery. Can J Surg 2012; 55(5):E8–9.
6. Lister J. On a new method of treating compound fracture, abscess, etc.: with observations on the conditions of suppuration. Lancet 1867;89(2272):326–9.
7. Koch R, Brock TD, Fred EB. The etiology of tuberculosis. Rev Infect Dis 1982; 4(6):1270–4.
8. Horan TC, Gaynes RP, Martone WJ, et al. CDC definitions of nosocomial surgical site infections, 1992: a modification of CDC definitions of surgical wound infections. Am J Infect Control 1992;20(5):271–4.
9. Riedel S, Hobden JA, Miller S, et al. Normal human microbiota. In: Weitz M, Thomas CM, editors. Jawetz, melnick, & adelberg's medical microbiology. 28th edition. New York: McGraw-Hill Education; 2019.
10. Davis CP. Normal flora. In: Baron S, editor. Medical microbiology. 4th edition. Galveston: University of Texas Medical Branch at Galveston; 1996.
11. Gillespie S, Bamford K. Medical microbiology and infection at a glance. Hoboken, (United Kingdom): John Wiley & Sons; 2012. Incorporated.
12. Miller JM, Binnicker MJ, Campbell S, et al. A guide to utilization of the microbiology laboratory for diagnosis of infectious diseases: 2018 update by the infectious diseases society of america and the american society for microbiologya. Clin Infect Dis 2018;67(6):e1–94.
13. Hidron AI, Edwards JR, Patel J, et al. NHSN annual update: antimicrobial-resistant pathogens associated with healthcare-associated infections: annual summary of data reported to the National healthcare safety network at the centers for disease control and prevention, 2006-2007. Infect Control Hosp Epidemiol 2008;29(11):996.

14. Stevens DL, Bisno AL, Chambers HF, et al. Practice guidelines for the diagnosis and management of skin and soft tissue infections: 2014 update by the infectious diseases society of America. Clin Infect Dis 2014;59(2):e10–52.

15. Pessaux P, Msika S, Atalla D, et al. Risk factors for postoperative infectious complications in noncolorectal abdominal surgery: a multivariate analysis based on a prospective multicenter study of 4718 patients. Arch Surg 2003;138(3):314–24.

16. Nolan MB, Martin DP, Thompson R, et al. Association between smoking status, preoperative exhaled carbon monoxide levels, and postoperative surgical site infection in patients undergoing elective surgery. JAMA Surg 2017;152(5): 476–83.

17. Hollenbeak CS, Lave JR, Zeddies T, et al. Factors associated with risk of surgical wound infections. Am J Med Qual 2006;21(6_suppl):29S–34S.

18. Sørensen LT. Wound healing and infection in surgery: the pathophysiological impact of smoking, smoking cessation, and nicotine replacement therapya systematic review. Ann Surg 2012;255(6):1069–79.

19. Culver DH, Horan TC, Gaynes RP, et al. Surgical wound infection rates by wound class, operative procedure, and patient risk index. Am J Med 1991;91(3, Supplement 2):S152–7.

20. Haley RW, Culver DH, Morgan WM, et al. Identifying patients at high risk of surgical wound infection: a simple multivariate index of patient susceptibility and wound contamination. Am J Epidemiol 1985;121(2):206–15.

21. Ortega G, Rhee DS, Papandria DJ, et al. An evaluation of surgical site infections by wound classification system using the ACS-NSQIP. J Surg Res 2012; 174(1):33–8.

22. Martone WJ, Nichols RL. Recognition, prevention, surveillance, and management of surgical site infections: introduction to the problem and symposium overview. Clin Infect Dis 2001;33(Supplement_2):S67–8.

23. CDC guidelines for the prevention and control of nosocomial infections. Guidelines for prevention of surgical wound infections, 1985. Am J Infect Control 1986;14(2):71.

24. Rubin RH. Surgical wound infection: epidemiology, pathogenesis, diagnosis and management. BMC Infect Dis 2006;6:171.

25. Tang R, Chen HH, Wang YL, et al. Risk factors for surgical site infection after elective resection of the colon and rectum: a single-center prospective study of 2,809 consecutive patients. Ann Surg 2001;234(2):181–9.

26. Anderson DJ, Podgorny K, Berríos-Torres SI, et al. Strategies to prevent surgical site infections in acute care hospitals: 2014 Update. Infect Control Hosp Epidemiol 2014;35(6):605–27.

27. Zimlichman E, Henderson D, Tamir O, et al. Health care–associated infections: a meta-analysis of costs and financial impact on the US health care system. JAMA Intern Med 2013;173(22):2039–46.

28. System NNIS. National Nosocomial Infections Surveillance (NNIS) system report, data summary from January 1992 through June 2004, issued October 2004. Am J Infect Control 2004;32:470–85.

29. Magill SS, O'Leary E, Janelle SJ, et al. Changes in prevalence of health care–associated infections in U.S. hospitals. N Engl J Med 2018;379(18):1732–44.

30. Magill SS, Edwards JR, Bamberg W, et al. Multistate point-prevalence survey of health care–associated infections. N Engl J Med 2014;370(13):1198–208.

31. McFarland A, Reilly J, Manoukian S, et al. The economic benefits of surgical site infection prevention in adults: a systematic review. J Hosp Infect 2020;106(1): 76–101.

32. Ban KA, Minei JP, Laronga C, et al. American college of surgeons and surgical infection society: surgical site infection guidelines, 2016 update. J Am Coll Surg 2017;224(1):59–74.

33. WHO Library Cataloguing-in-Publication Data Global Guidelines for the Prevention of Surgical Site Infection. World Health Organization; 2016.

34. Berrios S, Umscheid C, Bratzler D, et al. Centers for disease control and prevention guideline for the prevention of surgical site infection, 2017. JAMA Surg 2017; 152(8):784–91.

35. Fields AC, Pradarelli JC, Itani KMF. Preventing surgical site infections: looking beyond the current guidelines. JAMA 2020;323(11):1087–8.

36. Darouiche RO, Wall MJ Jr, Itani KM, et al. Chlorhexidine–alcohol versus povidone–iodine for surgical-site antisepsis. N Engl J Med 2010;362(1):18–26.

37. Stapleton EJ, Frane N, Lentz JM, et al. Association of disposable perioperative jackets with surgical site infections in a large multicenter health care organization. JAMA Surg 2020;155(1):15–20.

38. Wills BW, Smith WR, Arguello AM, et al. Association of surgical jacket and bouffant use with surgical site infection risk. JAMA Surg 2020;155(4):323–8.

39. Costa ML, Achten J, Knight R, et al. Effect of incisional negative pressure wound therapy vs standard wound dressing on deep surgical site infection after surgery for lower limb fractures associated with major trauma: the WHIST randomized clinical trial. JAMA 2020;323(6):519–26.

40. Matatov T, Reddy KN, Doucet LD, et al. Experience with a new negative pressure incision management system in prevention of groin wound infection in vascular surgery patients. J Vasc Surg 2013;57(3):791–5.

41. Shen P, Blackham AU, Lewis S, et al. Phase II randomized trial of negative-pressure wound therapy to decrease surgical site infection in patients undergoing laparotomy for gastrointestinal, pancreatic, and peritoneal surface malignancies. J Am Coll Surg 2017;224(4):726–37.

42. Loftus RW, Dexter F, Goodheart MJ, et al. The effect of improving basic preventive measures in the perioperative arena on staphylococcus aureus transmission and surgical site infections: a randomized clinical trial. JAMA Netw Open 2020; 3(3):e201934.

43. Bode LGM, Kluytmans JAJW, Wertheim HFL, et al. Preventing surgical-site infections in nasal carriers of staphylococcus aureus. N Engl J Med 2010;362(1):9–17.

44. Leaper DJ, Edmiston CE. World health organization: global guidelines for the prevention of surgical site infection. J Hosp Infect 2017;95(2):135–6.

45. Memtsoudis SG, Poeran J, Kehlet H. Enhanced recovery after surgery in the United States: from evidence-based practice to uncertain science? JAMA 2019;321(11):1049–50.

46. Hoang SC, Klipfel AA, Roth LA, et al. Colon and rectal surgery surgical site infection reduction bundle: To improve is to change. Am J Surg 2019;217(1):40–5.

47. Grant MC, Yang D, Wu CL, et al. Impact of enhanced recovery after surgery and fast track surgery pathways on healthcare-associated infections: results from a systematic review and meta-analysis. Ann Surg 2017;265(1):68–79.

48. Kummerow Broman K, Gaskill CE, Faqih A, et al. Evaluation of wound photography for remote postoperative assessment of surgical site infections. JAMA Surg 2019;154(2):117–24.

Overview of Aortic Stenosis

Rebecca Arko, MMSc, PA-C[a], Courtney Fankhanel, PA-C, MMSc[b],*

KEYWORDS

- Aortic stenosis • Aortic valve replacement • AVR

KEY POINTS

- Aortic stenosis (AS) is the most common valvular heart disease in the western world, accounting for 43% of all single, native, left-sided valve disease.
- Clinicians should be aware of the symptoms and physical examination findings patients may experience as a result of AS, as well as the appropriate management and escalation of care.
- Aortic valve replacement is the mainstay of treatment of significant aortic valve stenosis. This includes both surgical aortic valve replacement and transcatheter aortic valve replacement.

Aortic stenosis (AS) is the most common valvular heart disease in the western world, accounting for 43% of all single, native, left-sided valve disease.[1] The disease is more common in the elderly population and continues to increase in prevalence as the population ages. Consequently, the health care system must prepare for the growing number of patients with AS who necessitate an aortic valve replacement (AVR). Clinicians should be aware of the symptoms and physical examination findings patients may experience as a result of AS, as well as the appropriate management and escalation of care.

PREVALENCE

A meta-analysis found the prevalence of AS in the elderly (>75 years) to be 12.4%, with 3.4% of the population suffering from severe symptomatic AS (strong indication for intervention).[2] The younger population has considerably less disease, present in only about 5% of the population at the age of 65 years.[3] However, because of the degenerative nature of AS, which progresses with time, the prevalence of severe disease is considerably increasing. The number of cases in the elderly with an indication for surgery is projected to double by 2050, generating numerous ramifications on the health care system.[2]

[a] Cardiac Surgery, Yale New Haven Hospital, PO Box 208083, New Haven, CT 06520-8083, USA;
[b] Yale Physician Associate Program, PO Box 208083, New Haven, CT 06520-8083, USA
* Corresponding author.
E-mail address: courtney.fankhanel@yale.edu

Physician Assist Clin 6 (2021) 309–318
https://doi.org/10.1016/j.cpha.2020.11.004
2405-7991/21/© 2020 Elsevier Inc. All rights reserved.

physicianassistant.theclinics.com

PATHOGENESIS

Degenerative aortic valve calcification is the main mechanism of AS, accounting for 82% of AS valvulopathy. Degenerative AS has an insidious onset caused by atherosclerosis, calcification, and valve leaflet stiffening and remodeling, eventually progressing to obstruction of the left ventricular outflow. Degenerative AS progresses with age and patients commonly have multiple comorbidities. Additional risk factors are similar to those of atherosclerosis, such as smoking, hyperlipidemia, hypertension, diabetes, and elevated body mass index.[4] Rheumatic valve disease is the second most prevalent mechanism in the western world (11%); however, it accounts for most of the cases worldwide due to the greater prevalence of rheumatic disease globally. Congenital disease (bicuspid aortic valve) accounts for most of the remaining cases (5%).[5]

Bicuspid aortic valve is the most common congenital heart defect occurring in 0.5% to 2.0% of individuals.[6] The geometry of a bicuspid aortic valve causes mechanical stress and leads to premature calcification of the valve.[7] Patients with a bicuspid aortic valve usually need an AVR earlier in life with a mean age at the time of surgery around 50 years.[3] The presentation for these patients varies; some patients present symptomatically in infancy, whereas others are discovered much later in life with different sequela of the bicuspid valve (infectious endocarditis, aortopathy, AS).[8]

PATHOPHYSIOLOGY

The stiffening of the aortic valve leaflets causes the left ventricle to hypertrophy in order to maintain a normal cardiac output. This compensatory mechanism generally preserves left ventricular function while increasing the pressure gradient across the aortic valve. Ultimately, the left ventricle reaches a tipping point and systolic function declines due to the increased pressure required to overcome the left ventricular outflow tract. The pressure overload can lead to irreversible myocardial dysfunction.[9] However, with the proper intervention in a timely manner, some left systolic function can be recovered following AVR.[10]

The compensatory mechanism of left ventricular hypertrophy also leads to a decline in the ventricular compliance, resulting in increased diastolic pressures. These elevated filling pressures cause a backup on the left side of the heart, resulting in pulmonary edema and dyspnea. In addition, the coronary arteries are not able to supply the hypertrophic ventricle with adequate perfusion, consequently causing angina.

Angina is the result of a discrepancy between myocardial oxygen demand and supply, both of which have the potential to be negatively affected in AS. Increased systolic wall stress (due to the hypertrophic ventricle) increases oxygen demand. Meanwhile, increased filling pressures inside the ventricle decrease the supply.

Syncope results from a reduction in cerebral blood flow. In AS, systolic dysfunction with subsequent inadequate cranial perfusion leads to syncope. A heart with severe AS loses its ability to increase cardiac output with exercise, exacerbating these symptoms with physical activity.

SYMPTOMS

The classic symptoms of severe AS are dyspnea (50%), angina (35%), and syncope (15%), all of which are amplified with exertion.[10] Other patients present with ambiguous symptoms such as fatigue or a decrease in exercise tolerance. Regardless, progression to symptomatic AS is an important factor when determining severity and when to proceed with AVR. The presence of symptoms indicates an increased risk of sudden death with a life expectancy of only 3 years without AVR.[11] The average survival at the onset of angina, syncope, and dyspnea are 5, 3, and 2 years, respectively.[12] Event-free survival at 2 years has been found to be as low as 30%.[13] Because of the poor outcomes after the onset of symptoms, AVR should be considered for any patient with symptomatic AS.

Patients with AS have a low tolerance for atrial fibrillation because they rely on the atrial kick for maximum ventricular filling and subsequent cardiac output. Therefore, atrial fibrillation may exacerbate AS and patients may present earlier due to a lower compensatory response than similar patients without atrial fibrillation.

Patients with mild or moderate AS may present with similar symptoms; however, other causes of the symptoms should be considered. Many patients with AS have other comorbidities, which could play a larger role in the symptoms patients are experiencing. A broader differential is necessary in these patients to ensure that a different disease process is not being missed.

PHYSICAL EXAMINATION

The classic physical examination finding of AS is a harsh, crescendo-decrescendo, systolic murmur. It is heard best at the second intercostal space, right sternal boarder, and radiates to the carotids. As the severity of AS increases, the murmur peaks later and the duration extends. Occasionally, a fourth heart sound is appreciated due to the hypertrophic left ventricle. A slow and delayed carotid upstroke, along with a prolonged point of maximal impulse, may accompany the murmur. Elderly patients with severe vascular disease may have a near-normal physical examination, making the diagnosis more difficult in a clinical setting without the use of echocardiogram.

DIAGNOSTIC TESTING

Echocardiography is the primary tool used in diagnosing AS. A transthoracic echocardiogram (TTE) is an affordable and noninvasive test that can be completed on an outpatient basis. A TTE is indicated for any patient with new or worsening signs or symptoms of AS (class 1 recommendation).[14] TTE often shows a decreased aortic valve area (AVA), as well as thickening and calcification of the aortic valve. A TTE is used to determine valve anatomy and hemodynamics, left ventricular function, disease in other valves, pulmonary hypertension, and aortic root dilation.[15] The TTE evaluates the degree of disease severity, the size of the aortic valve and left ventricle, systolic function, and can help determine when an AVR is necessary.[14] Periodic monitoring with TTE is recommended every 6 months to 2 years, depending on the severity of disease (class 1 recommendation).[14]

As AS progresses, the AVA decreases and the velocity of flow across the valve generally increases. Doppler can be used to estimate the pressure gradient across the valve, the jet velocity, and AVA, which are pivotal in the staging of AS.[15] In addition, dobutamine stress echocardiography is used in patients with low-gradient AS to stage the disease and help determine interoperative risk during a surgical AVR.[16] Low-flow, low-gradient AS can result in underestimation of gradients and AVA measures using the traditional doppler testing, necessitating alternative measures such as low-dose dobutamine stress echocardiography.

Cardiac catheterization is used when there is a discrepancy between the patient's symptoms or physical examination findings and TTE. Catheterization allows for direct measurements of left ventricular and aortic pressures, as well as calculations of AVA and cardiac output.

Computed tomography and cardiac MRI are applied to a greater extent in the evaluation of aortic root and ascending aortic aneurysms. However, they have been used to assess valve calcification and anatomic aortic valve area.[10]

Exercise stress testing is useful in the assessment of asymptomatic but severe AS with a normal ejection fraction. Most of the patients with severe AS are older than 75 years and may have a more sedentary lifestyle due to other comorbidities and, therefore, will not exhibit symptoms. Others may attribute general fatigue and decreased stamina to the aging process. These patients may be asymptomatic even when objective data demonstrate severe AS. In these circumstances an exercise stress test can stimulate symptoms and indicate which patients need an AVR. An abnormal blood pressure response, symptoms of AS, exercise-induced arrythmias, and poor exercise capacity have been shown to correlate with poor 2-year symptom-free survival.[17] Consequently, patients with positive exercise stress tests should be evaluated for AVR.

Electrocardiography and chest radiography are not typically helpful in evaluating AS. Electrocardiography in patients with severe AS may demonstrate left ventricular hypertrophy or left atrial enlargement. Cardiomegaly and pulmonary edema on chest radiography are late signs of severe AS. In addition, a calcified aorta or aortic valve may be appreciated.

STAGING

The American College of Cardiology and American Heart Association have created a staging system that is used unanimously in the staging of valvular heart disease and AS (**Table 1**).[14] The primary factors in staging include the aortic valve area, maximum aortic jet velocity, and the aortic pressure gradient, all of which are calculated by echocardiogram. In addition to the objective data, the presence of symptoms influences staging.

Briefly, stage A patients are at risk of developing AS. This group includes patients with a bicuspid aortic valve or aortic sclerosis but who are asymptomatic with no hemodynamic changes. Stage B patients have progressive AS, which encompasses both mild and moderate AS. These patients have hemodynamic changes with elevated maximum aortic velocities (2.0–3.9 m/s) or pressure gradients (20–39 mm Hg). Stage C is reserved for patients with asymptomatic severe AS, with or without left ventricular dysfunction (Stage C2 and C1, respectively) and left ventricular hypertrophy. These patients have elevated maximum aortic velocities greater than 4 m/s, pressure gradients greater than 40 mm Hg, or AVA less than 1.0 cm². Stage C2 patients have a left ventricular ejection fraction of greater than 50%. Stage D is symptomatic severe AS and is divided into high-gradient, low-flow/low-gradient with reduced ejection fraction, and low-gradient with preserved ejection fraction (D1, D2, and D3 respectively). D1 has elevated maximum aortic velocities greater than 4 m/s, pressure gradients greater than 40 mm Hg, and AVA less than 1.0 cm². D2 and D3 have an AVA less than 1.0 cm²but with maximum aortic velocities less than 4 m/s or aortic pressure gradients less than 40 mm Hg.

MEDICAL MANAGEMENT

Patients with hypertension and concurrent asymptomatic AS or who are at risk for developing AS should be treated according to the guideline-directed medical therapy (class 1 recommendation). Statin therapy has demonstrated to be ineffective in slowing the progression of AS and therefore is not indicated for AS management (class III recommendation).[14] Other medical management has not been shown to be effective in treating or slowing the progression of AS. Therefore, surgical or transcatheter AVR is often indicated.

Table 1
Staging of aortic stenosis

Stage	Definition	Valve Anatomy	Valve Hemodynamics	Hemodynamic Consequences	Symptoms
A	At risk	• Bicuspid aortic valve (or other congenital valve anomaly) • Aortic valve sclerosis	Aortic V_{max} <2 m/s	None	None
B	Progressive	• Mild-to-moderate leaflet calcification of a bicuspid or trileaflet valve with some reduction in systolic motion or • Rheumatic valve changes with commissural fusion	• Mild AS: aortic V_{max} 2.0–2.9 m/s or mean ΔP <20 mm Hg • Moderate AS: aortic V_{max} 3.0–3.9 m/s or mean ΔP 20–39 mm Hg	• Early LV diastolic dysfunction may be present • Normal LVEF	None
C1	Asymptomatic severe	Severe leaflet calcification or congenital stenosis with severely reduced leaflet opening	• Aortic V_{max} ≥4 m/s or mean ΔP ≥40 mm Hg • AVA typically is ≤1.0 cm² (or AVAi ≤0.6 cm²/m²) • Very severe AS is an aortic V_{max} ≥5 m/s or mean ΔP ≥60 mm Hg	• LV diastolic dysfunction • Mild LV hypertrophy • Normal LVEF	None
C2	Asymptomatic severe with LV dysfunction	Severe leaflet calcification or congenital stenosis with severely reduced leaflet opening	• Aortic V_{max} ≥4 m/s or mean ΔP ≥40 mm Hg • AVA typically ≤1.0 cm² (or AVAi ≤0.6 cm²/m²)	LVEF <50%	None
D1	Symptomatic severe high-grade	Severe leaflet calcification or congenital stenosis with severely reduced leaflet opening	• Aortic V_{max} ≥4 m/s or mean ΔP ≥40 mm Hg • AVA typically ≤1.0 cm² (or AVAi ≤0.6 cm²/m²) but may be larger with mixed AS/AR	• LV diastolic dysfunction • LV hypertrophy • Pulmonary hypertension may be present	• Exertional dyspnea or decreased exercise tolerance • Exertional angina • Exertional syncope or presyncope

(continued on next page)

Table 1
(continued)

Stage	Definition	Valve Anatomy	Valve Hemodynamics	Hemodynamic Consequences	Symptoms
D2	Symptomatic severe low-flow with reduced LVEF	Severe leaflet calcification with severely reduced leaflet motion	• AVA $\leq$1.0 cm^2 with resting aortic V$_{max}$ <4 m/s or mean ΔP <40 mm Hg • Dobutamine stress echocardiography shows AVA $\leq$1.0 cm^2 with V$_{max}$ $\geq$4 m/s at any flow rate	• LV diastolic dysfunction • LV hypertrophy • LVEF <50%	• HF • Angina • Syncope or presyncope
D3	Symptomatic severe low-gradient with normal LVEF or paradoxic low-flow	Severe leaflet calcification with severely reduced leaflet motion	• AVA $\leq$1.0 cm^2 with aortic V$_{max}$ <4 m/s or mean ΔP <40 mm Hg • Indexed AVA $\leq$0.6 cm^2/m^2 and • Stroke volume index <35 mL/m^2 • Measured when patient is normotensive (systolic BP <140 mm Hg)	• Increased LV relative wall thickness • Small LV chamber with low stroke volume • Restrictive diastolic filling • LVEF $\geq$50%	• HF • Angina • Syncope or presyncope

Abbreviations: AR, aortic regurgitation; AVAi, aortic valve area indexed to body surface area; BP, blood pressure; HF, heart failure; LV, left ventricular; LVEF, left ventricular ejection fraction; V$_{max}$, maximum aortic velocity; ΔP, pressure gradient.

From Nishimura RA, Otto CM, Bonow RO, et al. 2014 AHA/ACC Guideline for the Management of Patients With Valvular Heart Disease: executive summary: a report of the American College of Cardiology/American Heart Association Task Force on Practice Guidelines. *Circulation.* 2014;129(23):2440-2492; with permission.

AORTIC VALVE REPLACEMENT

The lack of sufficient medical treatment has led to AVR as the mainstay of treatment of symptomatic patients and those with severe disease. As shown in **Fig. 1**, the guidelines broadly recommend that patients with severe AS and patients with mild-moderate AS undergoing other cardiac surgery should receive an AVR. AVR can be completed surgically or, more recently, with transcatheter AVR (TAVR). TAVR is a less invasive procedure often completed by an interventional cardiologist in a hybrid operating room. The recent advances seen with TAVR have given high-risk surgical patients a chance at AVR, which previously would not have been possible. Currently, TAVR is recommended for high- and intermediate-risk patients with ongoing studies about the long-term outcomes and utility in lower risk patients (**Fig. 2**).[18]

SURGICAL AORTIC VALVE REPLACEMENT

For most of the cardiac surgery history, surgical AVR (sAVR) was the only effective therapy for severe and/or symptomatic AS. With the introduction of TAVR, there now is an alternative in specific patient population cases; however, the field of sAVR continues to grow and innovate new techniques.

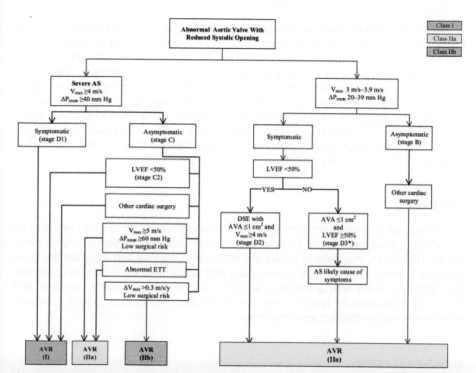

Fig. 1. Indications for aortic valve replacement. AS, aortic stenosis; AVA, aortic valve area; AVR, aortic valve replacement by either surgical or transcatheter approach; BP, blood pressure; DSE, dobutamine stress echocardiography; ETT, exercise treadmill test; LVEF, left ventricular ejection fraction; V_{max}, maximum velocity; ΔP_{mean}, mean pressure gradient. (*From* Nishimura RA, Otto CM, Bonow RO, et al. 2014 AHA/ACC Guideline for the Management of Patients With Valvular Heart Disease: executive summary: a report of the American College of Cardiology/American Heart Association Task Force on Practice Guidelines. *Circulation.* 2014;129(23):2440-2492; with permission.)

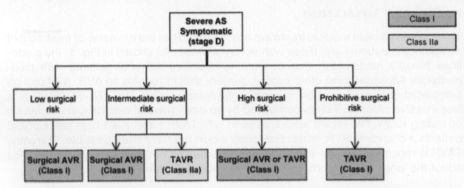

Fig. 2. Guidelines for transcatheter aortic valve replacement or surgical aortic valve replacement. AS, aortic stenosis; AVR, aortic valve replacement; TAVR, transcatheter aortic valve replacement. (*From* Nishimura RA, Otto CM, Bonow RO, et al. 2017 AHA/ACC Focused Update of the 2014 AHA/ACC Guideline for the Management of Patients With Valvular Heart Disease: A Report of the American College of Cardiology/American Heart Association Task Force on Clinical Practice Guidelines. *Circulation.* 2017;135(25):e1159-e1195.)

Traditional sAVR requires the use of the cardiopulmonary bypass machine to stop the heart to open the ascending aorta through an aortotomy to gain access to the aortic valve. Similar to many other forms of cardiac surgery, the traditional approach to exposing the heart is via median sternotomy. From a surgical exposure standpoint, sternotomy allows excellent access to the heart; however, it comes at the cost of disruption of the chest wall and longer recovery. Less invasive methods to perform sAVR include using a mini partial sternotomy approach[19] as well as a right mini thoracotomy approach.[20] Both of these minimally invasive approaches to sAVR still require the use of a cardiopulmonary bypass machine often times with alternative cannulation locations for the heart lung machine.

VALVE TYPES

When discussing valve replacement there are 2 main groupings of artificial valves used for sAVR. These categories include mechanical valves and tissue/bioprosthetic valves. Historically mechanical valves are considered durable and long-lasting; however, the primary disadvantage for many patients is the need for lifelong anticoagulation following sAVR with a mechanical valve. Tissue valves (bovine, porcine, and homografts) traditionally tend to degrade sooner than mechanical valves; however, they do not require lifelong anticoagulation.

CLINICS CARE POINTS

- Clinicians should look for the classic triad of symptoms of dyspnea, angina, and syncope when evaluating patients for aortic stenosis.
- When aortic stenosis is suspected based upon patient history, symptoms, or physical exam, transthoracic echocardiogram (TTE) should be ordered to evaluate the patient.
- If a patient has known aortic stenosis, periodic monitoring with TTE is recommended every 6 months to 2 years to evaluate the progression of the valvular disease.

DISCLOSURE

The authors have nothing to disclose.

REFERENCES

1. Iung B, Baron G, Butchart EG, et al. A prospective survey of patients with valvular heart disease in Europe: The Euro Heart Survey on Valvular Heart Disease. Eur Heart J 2003;24(13):1231–43.
2. Osnabrugge RLJ, Mylotte D, Head SJ, et al. Aortic stenosis in the elderly: disease prevalence and number of candidates for transcatheter aortic valve replacement: a meta-analysis and modeling study. J Am Coll Cardiol 2013;62(11):1002–12.
3. Ancona DR, Pinto DSC. Epidemiology of Aortic Valve Stenosis (AS) and of Aortic Valve Incompetence (AI): Is the Prevalence of AS/AI Similar in Different Parts of the World? Eur Soc Cardiol 2020;18(10).
4. Yan AT, Koh M, Chan KK, et al. Association between cardiovascular risk factors and aortic stenosis: The CANHEART Aortic Stenosis Study. J Am Coll Cardiol 2017;69(12):1523–32.
5. Carità P, Coppola G, Novo G, et al. Aortic stenosis: insights on pathogenesis and clinical implications. J Geriatr Cardiol 2016;13(6):489–98.
6. Coffey S, Cairns BJ, Iung B. The modern epidemiology of heart valve disease. Heart 2016;102(1):75.
7. Beppu S, Suzuki S, Matsuda H, et al. Rapidity of progression of aortic stenosis in patients with congenital bicuspid aortic valves. Am J Cardiol 1993;71(4):322–7.
8. Siu SC, Silversides CK. Bicuspid aortic valve disease. J Am Coll Cardiol 2010; 55(25):2789–800.
9. Bonow RO, Carabello BA, Chatterjee K, et al. 2008 Focused update incorporated into the ACC/AHA 2006 guidelines for the management of patients with valvular heart disease: a report of the American College of Cardiology/American Heart Association Task Force on Practice Guidelines (Writing Committee to Revise the 1998 Guidelines for the Management of Patients With Valvular Heart Disease): endorsed by the Society of Cardiovascular Anesthesiologists, Society for Cardiovascular Angiography and Interventions, and Society of Thoracic Surgeons. Circulation 2008;118(15):e523–661.
10. Maganti K, Rigolin VH, Sarano ME, et al. Valvular heart disease: diagnosis and management. Mayo Clin Proc 2010;85(5):483–500.
11. Bach DS, Siao D, Girard SE, et al. Evaluation of patients with severe symptomatic aortic stenosis who do not undergo aortic valve replacement: the potential role of subjectively overestimated operative risk. Circ Cardiovasc Qual Outcomes 2009; 2(6):533–9.
12. Braunwald E. Aortic Stenosis. Circulation 2018;137(20):2099–100.
13. Rosenhek R, Binder T, Porenta G, et al. Predictors of outcome in severe, asymptomatic aortic stenosis. N Engl J Med 2000;343(9):611–7.
14. Nishimura RA, Otto CM, Bonow RO, et al. 2014 AHA/ACC Guideline for the Management of Patients With Valvular Heart Disease: executive summary: a report of the American College of Cardiology/American Heart Association Task Force on Practice Guidelines. Circulation 2014;129(23):2440–92.
15. Baumgartner H, Otto CM. Aortic stenosis severity: do we need a new concept? J Am Coll Cardiol 2009;54(11):1012–3.
16. Kanwar A, Thaden JJ, Nkomo VT. Management of patients with aortic valve stenosis. Mayo Clin Proc 2018;93(4):488–508.

17. Amato MC, Moffa PJ, Werner KE, et al. Treatment decision in asymptomatic aortic valve stenosis: role of exercise testing. Heart 2001;86(4):381–6.

18. Nishimura RA, Otto CM, Bonow RO, et al. 2017 AHA/ACC Focused Update of the 2014 AHA/ACC Guideline for the Management of Patients With Valvular Heart Disease: A Report of the American College of Cardiology/American Heart Association Task Force on Clinical Practice Guidelines. Circulation 2017;135(25): e1159–95.

19. Benetti FJ, Mariani MA, Rizzardi JL, et al. Minimally invasive aortic valve replacement. J Thorac Cardiovasc Surg 1997;113(4):806–7.

20. Gundry SR, Shattuck OH, Razzouk, et al. Facile minimally invasive cardiac surgery via ministernotomy. Ann Thorac Surg 1998;65(4):1100–4.

Chronic Venous Insufficiency

Bri Kestler, PA-C, MMS

KEYWORDS

- Venous insufficiency • Valvular incompetence • Venous duplex • Varicose veins
- Compression therapy • Sclerotherapy • Endovenous ablation

KEY POINTS

- Chronic venous insufficiency is a common vascular disorder in which valvular incompetence or venous pump dysfunction generates venous hypertension.
- Early disease manifests as leg pain, edema, and bulging varicosities, with skin changes and ulcer formation in advanced disease.
- Venous duplex provides noninvasive office-based diagnosis, and classification systems are available to aide in disease progression monitoring and treatment response.
- Compression therapy is a cornerstone of treatment and aides in countering the increased hydrostatic venous pressures caused by valvular incompetence.
- Sclerotherapy and endovenous thermal ablation trigger an inflammatory response that leads to fibrosis and closure of dysfunctional venous segments.

INTRODUCTION

Chronic venous insufficiency (CVI) is the most common vascular disorder in the world with more than 25 million adults in the United States afflicted with varicose veins, and more than 6 million with advanced venous disease.[1,2] CVI describes a condition that has many risk factors and cultivates in persistent ambulatory venous hypertension. Various pathologies occur because of changes within the venous system, with the most common clinical manifestations including leg pain, edema, and skin changes. Advanced venous disease is complicated by the presence of hyperpigmentation, cutaneous ulcers, and venous eczema. Socioeconomic consequences of CVI include impaired social engagement, loss of work hours because of disabling symptoms, diminished quality of life, and financial burden to patients and the health care system.[1]

OVERVIEW OF VENOUS PHYSIOLOGY

Oxygenated blood flows out of the left heart and eventually enters a microcirculatory environment that includes metarterioles, precapillary sphincters, and capillary beds.

Simulation Program, University of South Alabama, 5741 USA Drive North, Mobile, AL 36688-0002, USA
E-mail address: bri.kestler@gmail.com

Physician Assist Clin 6 (2021) 319–330
https://doi.org/10.1016/j.cpha.2020.11.005
2405-7991/21/© 2020 Elsevier Inc. All rights reserved.

Precapillary sphincters are naturally closed and open in response to oxygen and nutritional requirements of surrounding tissues. After exchange of gases and substances occurs between the blood and interstitial fluid, multiple capillaries join to create a postcapillary venule and eventually a vein. Veins have larger diameters and thinner walls than arteries, which allow more blood to flow with less vascular resistance. These anatomic differences allow veins to perform their functions as a reservoir to store blood and a conduit to return blood to the heart.

Superficial veins are located above the deep muscular fascia and include the truncal veins (greater and smaller saphenous) and numerous accessory veins. Perforators veins provide communication between the superficial and deep systems, with deep veins collecting blood and draining it from the extremity. Deep veins are located beneath the muscular fascia and lie within or between muscles. Deep veins are also called intermuscular veins; typically run in tandem with the arteries; and include the anterior and posterior tibial, peroneal, popliteal, and femoral veins.

Extremity veins contain bicuspid, one-way valves to assist in maintaining unidirectional flow of blood, especially in an upright position where increased effects of gravity are noted.[1] The valves open to allow blood to enter a vein segment, and then close to prevent retrograde blood flow. The number of valves within a vein segment increases in direct relation to hydrostatic pressures, with the distal leg containing the greatest number of valves. Competent valves prevent transmission of blood flow back into the capillaries, which would lead to increased leakage of blood products into the interstitium and tissue damage.

Another important component of the venous system is the venous pump. This involves contraction of leg muscles, primarily in the calf, to increase the subfascial pressure above the intramuscular vein pressures and propel venous blood into the deep system. The combination of competent valves and an effective venous pump ensures adequate return of venous blood, against gravity, to the right heart.

PATHOGENESIS OF VENOUS DISEASE

Valvular incompetence is the most common cause of venous hypertension and occurs within the deep, perforator, and/or superficial veins.

- Deep valvular dysfunction is most often the consequence of damage from a previous deep vein thrombosis (DVT). Rapid refilling of the deep veins, by retrograde flow, reduces the amount of blood drained from the extremity, and rapidly elevates pressures if the venous pump is not activated.
- Failure of perforator valves allows high pressure to enter the superficial system, leading to distention of superficial veins and secondary failure of the valves.
- Superficial valvular dysfunction allows retrograde blood flow, or reflux, into the microcirculation leading to increased hydrostatic pressures.[2] Incompetence of superficial valves has been shown in almost 90% of patients presenting with CVI, with reflux of the greater saphenous vein accounting for 70% to 80% of those patients.[1]

Venous pump dysfunction leads to ineffective emptying of venous blood from the distal legs and rapid elevation of postambulatory venous pressures. Rarely is venous pump dysfunction the primary cause of venous hypertension, but may occur with neuromuscular conditions or muscle-wasting syndromes.[1]

Venous hypertension produces cellular changes that weaken venous walls, leading to the development of venous microangiopathy. Dilation and tortuosity of veins is caused by a reduction in the number of smooth muscle cells in venous walls, and thickening of basement membranes with increased collagen and elastic fibers.[1] As venous and capillary pressures become high, endothelial damage with widening of interendothelial spaces and degradation of extracellular matrix leads to increased vascular permeability.[3] Capillary walls are normally permeable to allow for exchange of nutrients and waste products, but increased pressures lead to inadequate diffusion of nutritional materials and excessive fluid entering the interstitial tissue.

Risk factors for CVI are divided into primary and secondary factors (**Table 1**) and revolve around the concept that damage of the valves or loss of the venous pump will lead to chronic venous hypertension. CVI risk increases during pregnancy because of two mechanisms. First, the growing uterus compresses the iliac veins, creating a venous outflow stenosis/obstruction. Limited outflow leads to increased venous pressures with muscle contraction, venous engorgement, and failure of deep vein valves. Second, normal valves become excessively distensible under the influence of pregnancy hormones.[2] A family history of varicose veins is present in more than one-third of patients.[4]

Occupational risk is associated with prolonged periods of standing or sitting, because this disengages the venous pump causing blood to collect in the veins leading to increased pressures. To accommodate for the increase in pressure, the thin walled veins begin to dilate. Short periods of venous distention does not damage the valves, but chronic dilation causes the valvular leaflets to pull away from each other, leading to compromised function and incomplete closure. Historically, an estimated three-fold female predominance of CVI existed, yet more recent studies have shown similar risk among genders when corrected for age.[1,5,6] Secondary risk factors, such as DVT, phlebitis, or trauma to the vein from a lower extremity injury, leads to inappropriate venous repair and damage to the venous walls.

CLINICAL MANIFESTATIONS

Symptoms associated with CVI are vague and variable, and the same clinical manifestations result from different causes of disease. Typical pain is characterized as an aching, tight or heavy feeling that is worse after long periods of standing and is relieved with leg elevation.[2,4] Leg discomfort is thought to be caused by increased intracompartmental and subcutaneous volume and pressure.[1] Legs fatigue easily and patients with disease of the deep system may develop intense leg pain with ambulation, also known as venous claudication. Paresthesia is typically described as burning or electrical like pains, or a crawling sensation.[4]

Physical examination findings occur because of alterations of the venous walls and valves, causing abnormal venous architecture and skin changes, caused by increased permeability of the veins. It is important to have the patient standing while performing

Table 1 Chronic venous insufficiency risk factors	
Primary Risk Factors	**Secondary Risk Factors**
Pregnancy	Venous thrombi/phlebitis
Family history of varicose veins	Lower extremity trauma
Occupational risk	
Age	
Obesity	
Female gender	

the physical examination to maximize venous distention. Edema is typically pitting, forms with longer periods of standing, and generally begins in the malleolar region.

Alterations to Venous Network

- Spider veins are clusters of tiny blood vessels that develop close to the surface of the skin. They are often red, blue, or purple; and they have the appearance of a spiderweb or fan.
- Reticular veins are 2 to 3 mm in diameter and a bright blue or purple color. They typically present on the inner thighs or calves, and the back of the legs. Reticular veins do not protrude above the surface of the skin as much as varicose veins.
- Varicose veins are dilated superficial veins that bulge and take on a tortuous course under the skin. Varicosities are soft to palpation and may become painful as dilation increases. Varicose veins are differentiated from reticular veins by their increased size and lack of color, although larger varicose veins that push to the surface appear blue. Smaller varicosities may develop superficial thrombophlebitis with tenderness, erythema, and induration along the course of the vein. Palpation of the lower extremities detects additional varicosities that were not readily apparent on inspection. Varicose veins located over boney prominences are more susceptible to rupture.[7]

Skin Changes

- Red to brown hyperpigmentation caused by hemosiderin deposition occurs in diffuse patches or circumferentially in advanced disease. Erythematous and scaly patches of skin on the distal legs, or eczematous dermatitis, tends to be pruritic and is caused by chronic edema and interstitial cellular debris.[7]
- Lipodermatosclerosis results from activated leukocytes entering interstitial tissue and releasing proinflammatory cytokines that damage vascular walls. Fibrotic remodeling of the dermis and subcutaneous fat takes place, leading to chronic erythema and firm induration.
- Cutaneous ulcers are formed by proteolytic enzymes entering the interstitial tissue and degrading extracellular matrix and dermal structures. Venous ulcers tend to be shallow, cobblestoned in appearance, and irregular in shape.[2] Active and healed ulcers, typically in a distribution near the medial ankle with greater saphenous involvement or lateral ankle with smaller saphenous disease, are more common with advanced disease or comorbid conditions.

The Brodie-Trendelenburg test is performed at the bedside and helps distinguish valvular incompetence between the greater saphenous and perforator/deep veins. The test is performed by laying the patient on an examination table in a supine position and elevating the leg to drain the superficial veins. A tourniquet or manual compression is applied close to the groin along the superficial system, the patient is moved into an upright position, and the leg is inspected. A compromised perforator or deep system causes varicose veins to dilate rapidly (<20 seconds), whereas superficial disease takes more than 20 seconds to manifest protruding varicosities.[1,4] The Brodie-Trendelenburg test is 91% sensitive for superficial and perforator reflux, although poorly specific (15%).[4]

DIAGNOSTIC STUDIES

The most common initial study to diagnose CVI is a venous duplex study, which combines two-dimensional visualization to measure the diameter of dilated veins, and a pulsed Doppler assessment of flow direction.[1] A venous duplex study begins with the patient in a supine position, with the hip externally rotated and the knee flexed, to evaluate the deep system.[4] Venous patency is assessed via compression by the transducer, and multiple maneuvers assist in appraising venous flow patterns. Valvular competence is evaluated with the patient in a reverse Trendelenburg position and Valsalva maneuvers for upper thigh segments and caudal calf compression for lower limb segments.[2,4]

A more sensitive maneuver involves applying a blood pressure cuff to a patient's calf and rapidly inflating and deflating it with the patient in an upright position[8]; this is also beneficial because one method is used to study all the limb veins.[4] Reflux is defined as more than 0.5 seconds of reverse flow in superficial veins and/or more than 1 second of reverse flow in deep veins.[2,9] Reflux may be present in isolated segments or over the entire course of a vein. Additional tests, such as venography, venous pressure measurements, and/or plethysmography, should be reserved for patients with ambiguous findings on venous duplex.[2,4]

CLASSIFICATION SYSTEMS

Initial attempts to classify CVI focused solely on clinical appearance and led to lack of diagnostic precision and inability to reproduce treatment results. The Clinical, Etiology, Anatomic, Pathophysiology (CEAP) classification scheme was created by the American Venous Forum in 1994 to provide uniformity in the diagnosing and reporting of CVI.[1,4,10] Each category is broken down into subidentifiers to provide patients with an objective evaluation to be used as a marker for disease progression and/or improvement after therapy (**Table 2**).

A three-part Venous Severity Score to complement CEAP classification was created and is an easy and useful tool to evaluate response to treatment.[4,11] The Venous Severity Score includes the Venous Clinical Severity Score, Venous Segmental Disease Score, and Venous Disability Score.

- The Venous Clinical Severity Score (**Table 3**) involves 10 elements, each graded on a severity scale (absent, mild, moderate, or severe) and is best if jointly

Table 2
CEAP classification

Clinical Classification (C)	Etiologic Classification (E)
C_0 - no visible sign of disease	E_C - congenital
C_1 - spider veins, telangiectasias, or reticular veins	E_P - primary E_s - secondary
C_2 - varicose veins	E_N - no venous cause identified
C_3 - varicose veins with edema	Anatomic Classification (A)
C_{4a} - varicose veins with pigmentation or eczema	A_S - superficial veins A_P - perforator veins
C_{4b} - varicose veins with lipodermatosclerosis or atrophie blanche	A_D - deep veins A_O - no location identified
C_5 - healed venous ulcer	Pathophysiologic Classification (P)
C_6 - active venous ulcer	P_R - reflux
SUBSCRIPT	P_O - obstruction
S - symptomatic	$P_{R,O}$ - reflux and obstruction
A - asymptomatic	P_N - no pathophysiology identified

Table 3
Venous clinical severity score

Element	None = 0	Mild = 1	Moderate = 2	Severe = 3
Pain (or other discomfort)		Occasional pain that does not restrict regular daily activity	Daily pain that is interfering but does not prevent regular daily activity	Daily pain that limits most regular daily activities
Varicose veins (≥3 mm in diameter in standing position)		Few, scattered (isolated branch varicosities or clusters)	Confined to calf or thigh	Involves calf and thigh
Venous edema		Limited to foot and ankle area	Extends above ankle but below knee	Extends to knee and above
Skin pigmentation (does not include focal pigmentation over varicose veins)		Limited to perimalleolar area	Diffuse over lower third of calf	Wider distribution above lower third of calf
Inflammation (erythema, cellulitis, venous eczema, dermatitis)		Limited to perimalleolar area	Diffuse over lower third of calf	Wider distribution above lower third of calf
Induration (includes atrophie blanche and lipodermato-sclerosis)		Limited to perimalleolar area	Diffuse over lower third of calf	Wider distribution above lower third of calf
Active ulcer number	0	1	2	≥3
Active ulcer duration (longest active)	N/A	<3 mo	>3 mo but <1 y	Not healed for >1 y
Active ulcer size (largest active)	N/A	Diameter <2 cm	Diameter 2–6 cm	Diameter >6 cm
Compression therapy	Not used	Intermittent use of hose	Wears hose most days	Full compliance; wears hose every day

Abbreviation: N/A, non-applicable

completed by the clinician and the patient.[1,10] There is a maximum score of 30 points.

- The Venous Segmental Disease Score (**Table 4**) combines the anatomic and pathophysiologic portions of the CEAP and grades major venous segments according to presence of reflux and/or obstruction, based on venous duplex

Table 4
Venous segmental disease score

			Greater Saphenous (only if from Groin
0.5	Smaller Saphenous Thrombosed	1	to Below knee)
1	Greater saphenous	1	Calf veins, multiple
0.5	Perforators, thigh	2	Popliteal vein
1	Perforators, calf	1	Superficial femoral vein
2	Calf veins, multiple (posterior tibial vein alone = 1)	1	Profunda femoris vein
2	Popliteal vein	2	Common femoral vein
1	Superficial femoral vein	1	Iliac vein
1	Profunda femoris vein	1	Inferior vena cava
1	Common femoral vein and above		

studies. The Venous Segmental Disease Score weighs 11 venous segments for their relative importance when involved with reflux and/or obstruction.[10] There is a maximum of 10 points for either reflux and obstruction.

- The Venous Disability Score (**Table 5**) incorporates patient symptoms, ability to participate in activities of daily living, and their need for compression therapy. Usual activities refer to normal activities carried out before being disabled because of venous disease.[10]

TREATMENT
Conservative Therapy

Initial treatment of venous insufficiency includes lifestyle changes; modifications of risk factors; and compression hose to diminish symptoms, slow disease progression, and prevent complications. Leg elevation performed three to four times a day, for 30 minutes at a time, uses gravity to move extra blood volume from the superficial veins into the deep veins. Increased lower extremity activity includes light walking, or plantar flexion and heel lift exercises from a seated position.

Compression therapy offers external pressure to the lower extremities to counter the hydrostatic forces of venous hypertension.[1,2] Compression hose come in a variety of styles, from knee highs to full pantyhose varieties that come up to the waist. Compression hose available over the counter have a constant pressure gradient typically less than 20 mm Hg. Prescription compression hose are available in multiple strength intervals including 15 to 20 mm Hg, 20 to 30 mm Hg, 30 to 40 mm Hg, and

Table 5
Venous disability score

Score	Parameters
0	Asymptomatic
1	Symptomatic but able to carry out usual activities without compression therapy
2	Can carry out usual activities only with compression therapy and/or limb elevation
3	Unable to carry out usual activities even with compression therapy and/or limb elevation

40 to 50 mm Hg. Prescribed tensions are based on clinical severity with 20 to 30 mm Hg for CEAP classes C_2 to C_3, 30 to 40 mm Hg for C_4 to C_6, and 40 to 50 mm Hg for recurrent ulcers.[1,2] Prescription compression hose use a variable pressure gradient where the pressure at the toe is greater than the pressure at the top of the hose. Compression hose should be changed out every 6 to 9 months, if worn daily, because the elastic begins to breakdown and the tension supplied decreases.

A clinician should take into consideration patient comorbidities and feasibility of use, before prescribing compression hose. Hand arthritis, muscular atrophy, orthopedic injuries, and/or body habitus make application of higher strength compression hose difficult and assistive devices make donning easier. Compression hose assistive devices include wire structures that the patient prestretches the compression hose around, and then steps into the device and uses handles to pull the whole structure up their leg. Other devices have the patient wrap the hose around a thick elastic ring, step into the ring, and apply the hose as they unroll the ring up their leg. Doffing aides are also available for patients who have difficulty removing compression hose. Patients with coexisting peripheral arterial disease should be evaluated by a vascular specialist, to ensure compression therapy will not lead to complications because of arterial hypoperfusion.

Patients with arterial disease or cutaneous ulcers benefit from multilayer compression wraps, because they are lighter compression, and assist in wound healing through absorption of fluid. A traditional three-layer wrap comprises a padded first layer, conforming second layer involving a high-stretch bandage, and a short-stretch bandage to create a compressive third layer. All layers are applied in a spiral fashion, starting distal and moving proximal with a 50% overlap. Layers one and two are applied without any stretch, and layer three is applied with moderate stretch. These same principles are used when applying a two- or four-layer wrap, with changes to the composition of each layer. Medicated forms of compression wraps include an initial layer of gauze, impregnated with either zinc, glycerin, or calamine, being applied directly to the skin before application of additional layers.

Sclerotherapy

Lifestyle changes and compression hose provide symptomatic relief of venous insufficiency but do not change the abnormalities within the venous architecture. Referral to a vascular specialist is warranted if conservative therapy has failed or has not provided satisfactory results, or their CEAP class is C_4 to C_6.[1] Vascular specialists perform a variety of venous procedures for advanced treatment of CVI. Most insurance companies require a 90-day trial of compression therapy before paying for more invasive management strategies.

Sclerotherapy is the injection of a sclerosing agent, such as sodium tetradecyl sulfate, polidocanol, glycerin, and sodium morrhuate.[2,11] Injection of a sclerosant agent into a diseased vein causes irritation, inflammation, and eventual closure of the vein. Surrounding veins with competent anatomy then take up the venous burden and appropriately move it to the deep system. Sclerotherapy is effective for closure of spider, reticular, and superficial varicose veins. Common complications include hyperpigmentation along the course of the sclerosed vein, caused by hemosiderin deposition into the surrounding tissue, postinjection phlebitis, and postinjection pain.[1,2,12]

Interventional Procedures

Procedures using thermal energy in the form of radiofrequency (RF) or laser are used to ablate incompetent truncal veins or combined superficial/perforator disease.

Endovenous ablation begins with tumescent anesthesia, consisting of saline mixed with sodium bicarbonate and lidocaine, injected into the perivenous fascia along the course of the affected vein. Tumescent anesthesia prevents the overlying skin from thermal burns and reduces pain allowing for earlier return to normal activities.[1,2] Ultrasound identifies the affected vein and after a sheath is positioned, an endovenous thermal energy catheter is introduced. The catheter is advanced to the proximal point of insufficiency, typically the saphenofemoral junction, under ultrasound guidance. Once in position, the catheter is activated, and heat generated creates a local thermal injury to the venous wall, leading to inflammation, thrombosis, and fibrosis.[1,2,7] Continued activation of the catheter provides injury to the diseased venous segment as the catheter is slowly removed, leading to collapse of the incompetent vein.

Both ablation techniques carry high success rates, with 85% of patients receiving RF ablation of the greater saphenous vein demonstrating complete obliteration after 2 years.[13] Thermal ablation with laser energy has a complete saphenous closure success rate of 93% after 2 years.[14] Studies comparing RF and laser ablation revealed that RF ablation was associated with less postoperative pain and bruising.[15–17] Other common complications after thermal ablation include thrombophlebitis, hyperpigmentation, hematoma, skin burns, and cutaneous nerve injury.[7] Endovenous ablation is performed under moderate sedation in an outpatient setting. Postoperative instructions include increased leg elevation for 2 to 3 days, daily compression hose use for 1 to 2 weeks, and nonsteroidal anti-inflammatory drugs for pain. A follow-up venous duplex study is performed 2 days postoperatively to evaluate for vein closure and DVT. Valvular incompetence of the truncal veins leads to reflux into the superficial veins and increased dilation of varicosities. Closure of the truncal veins cause superficial varicosities to diminish in appearance, and therefore saphenous veins should be treated before sclerotherapy of superficial veins.

Ligation and stripping of truncal veins prevent reflux into the superficial system through interruption of flow and removal of diseased vein. Greater saphenous ligation and stripping has been the historical treatment of CVI, but has fallen out of favor because of longer recovery times; higher recurrence rates; and increased risk of typical surgical complications, such as hematoma, cellulitis, and abscess formation.[7] Studies comparing endovenous ablation with conventional ligation and stripping found that short-term efficacy between the two are comparable, but 3-year closure rates were 84% with RF ablation, 94% with laser ablation, and 78% with surgical ligation and stripping.[18] Thermal ablations also demonstrated improved quality of life and earlier return to normal activities and work, when compared with surgical stripping.[19,20]

Perforator disease contributes to ulcer formation, skin breakdown, and fibrotic changes. This makes accessing the local perforator responsible for the elevated venous pressures and manifestations difficult. Subfascial endoscopic surgery allows the diseased perforator vein to be accessed and ligated from a distant location, but conflicting data question this procedure's benefit. Treatment of local perforator disease is recommended in patients with CEAP class C_5 to C_6, with recent studies favoring endovenous ablation and foam sclerotherapy over the more invasive subfascial endoscopic surgery.[11]

Novel Ablative Techniques

Newer ablative techniques that have gained Food and Drug Administration approval include sclerosant foam, endovenous chemical adhesive, and a combined mechanical occlusion with chemical assistance (MOCA) device.[7] Nonthermal methods are used as monotherapy or adjunct treatment to endovenous ablations.

- Polidocanol microfoam (Varithena) combines polidocanol with a gas combination of 65% oxygen, 35% carbon dioxide, and a trace of nitrogen. Foam sclerotherapy, performed under ultrasound guidance, has demonstrated efficacy for closure of the greater and/or smaller saphenous veins.[12] Foam sclerotherapy offers a recovery time similar to endovenous ablations, but carries a higher rate of technical failure compared with thermal procedures.[21]
- Cyanoacrylate glue (VenaSeal) is a liquid adhesive that solidifies on contact with blood products, triggering an inflammatory response, fibrosis, and vein closure. Small amounts of the adhesive are delivered into the refluxing vein via a specialized endovenous catheter, followed by external compression, which physically closes the vein in short segments at a time. Early studies have demonstrated 92% 1-year closure rates of the greater saphenous vein after VenaSeal application.[22,23]
- ClariVein is a MOCA instrument that uses an endovenous wire rotating at 3500 rotations per minute to injure the venous wall. As the wire is spinning the MOCA catheter simultaneously injects a liquid sclerosant.[7] Two-year study results comparing greater saphenous vein closure showed lower success rates with the ClariVein (80%) when compared with RF ablation (88.3%).[24]

Deep System Management

Valvular incompetence within the deep system cannot be treated with thermal or chemical ablation, because of the critical role it plays in return of blood to the heart. Patients with lower CEAP classes have traditionally been treated with lifestyle changes and compression therapy, with valve reconstruction reserved for advanced CVI with recurrent ulcers and disabling symptoms.[1] Open and closed valvuloplasty techniques for venous repair are available, with more specialized procedures performed when valve destruction is caused by thrombotic etiologies.

Venous outflow stenosis in the deep system, particularly the iliac veins, leads to severe CVI and increased risk of ulcer formation. Stenosis/obstruction of the deep system is treated through endovenous angioplasty and stent placement to restore venous outflow. Efficacy of stenting procedures has increased to the point that it is an alternative to an open surgical venous bypass surgery.[2] Endovenous vein stenting mitigates the outflow obstruction and leads to relief of pain in approximately 50%, resolution of edema in 30%, and healing of ulcers in 50% of patients with iliac vein stenosis.[25]

SUMMARY

Competent valves and an effective venous pump are required for adequate return of venous blood to the heart. Dysfunction or alteration of normal physiology allows for development of venous hypertension and CVI. A variety of manifestations exist, with more advanced disease presenting with hyperpigmentation, lipodermatosclerosis, and venous ulcers. The treatment of CVI is based on the intensity of clinical manifestations, location, and cause of disease, and is guided with the use of classification scoring schemes. Compression therapy is the foundation of conservative management and provides symptomatic relief caused by reduction of hydrostatic venous pressures. Endovenous surgical interventions have become more common than traditional ligation and stripping, because of faster recovery times and lower recurrence rates. Newer ablative techniques use nonthermal approaches, such as foam sclerosant, chemical adhesives, and combined mechanical/chemical instruments, for closure of incompetent veins.

CLINICS CARE POINTS

- Physical exam should involve the patient standing, to maximize venous distention, and palpation of the lower extremities, to identify varicosities not readily apparent.
- Compression stockings should be prescribed after the initial visit, with a follow up visit in 90 days to reassess clinical manifestations and efficacy of therapy.
- Progression of the disease involves increases in hyperpigmentation, malleolar edema, and ulcer formation.
- Endovenous laser ablation carries a high success rate for treatment of truncal venous insufficiency, with radio frequency ablation specifically having less postoperative pain and bruising.

DISCLOSURE

The author denies any commercial or financial conflicts of interest or funding sources for the formation of this article.

REFERENCES

1. Eberhardt RT, Raffetto JD. Chronic venous insufficiency. Circulation 2014;130(4): 333–46.
2. Hyder O, Soukas P. Chronic venous insufficiency: novel management strategies for an under-diagnosed disease process. R I Med J 2017;100(5):37–9.
3. Gschwandtner ME, Ehringer H. Microcirculation in chronic venous insufficiency. Vasc Med 2001;6:169–79.
4. Krishnan S, Nicholls S. Chronic venous insufficiency: clinical assessment and patient selection. Semin Intervent Radiol 2005;22(3):169–77.
5. Ruckley C, Evans CJ, Allan PL, et al. Chronic venous insufficiency: clinical and duplex correlations: the Edinburgh Vein study of venous disorders in the general population. J Vasc Surg 2002;36:520–5.
6. Cesarone MR, Belcaro G, Nicolaides AN, et al. "Real" epidemiology of varicose veins and chronic venous diseases: the San Valentino vascular screening project. Angiology 2002;53(2):119–30.
7. Agrawal S, Saber W. Venous ablation. Interv Cardiol Clin 2020;9(2):255–63.
8. Markel A, Meissner MH, Manzo RA, et al. A comparison of the cuff deflation method with Valsalva's maneuver and limb compression in detecting venous valvular reflux. Arch Surg 1994;129(7):701–5.
9. Labropoulos N, Tiongson J, Pryor L, et al. Definition of venous reflux in lower-extremity veins. J Vasc Surg 2003;38:793–8.
10. Rutherford RB, Padberg FT, Comerota AJ, et al. Venous severity scoring: an adjunct to venous outcome assessment. J Vasc Surg 2000;31(6):1307–12.
11. Gloviczki P, Comerota AJ, Dalsing MC, et al. The care of patients with varicose veins and associated chronic venous diseases: clinical practice guidelines of the Society for Vascular Surgery and the American Venous Forum. J Vasc Surg 2011;53(5):2S–48S.
12. Memetoglu M, Yilmaz M, Kehlibar T, et al. Ultrasonography-guided foam sclerotherapy in patients with small saphenous vein insufficiency. J Vasc Surg Venous Lymphat Disord 2020;8(5):799–804.
13. Merchant RF, Depalma RG, Kabnick LS, et al. Endovascular obliteration of saphenous reflux: a multicenter study. J Vasc Surg 2002;35:1190–6.

14. Min RJ, Khilnani N, Zimmet SE. Endovenous laser treatment of saphenous vein reflux: long-term results. J Vasc Interv Radiol 2003;14(8):991–6.
15. Nordon IM, Hinchliffe RJ, Brar R, et al. A prospective double-blind randomized controlled trial of radiofrequency versus laser treatment of the great saphenous vein in patients with varicose veins. Ann Surg 2011;254(6):876–81.
16. Shepherd AC, Gohel MS, Brown LC, et al. Randomized clinical trial of VNUS® ClosureFASTTM radiofrequency ablation versus laser for varicose veins. Br J Surg 2010;97(6):810–8.
17. Goode SD, Chowdhury A, Crockett M, et al. Laser and radiofrequency ablation study (LARA study): a randomised study comparing radiofrequency ablation and endovenous laser ablation (810nm). Eur J Vasc Endovasc Surg 2010; 40(2):246–53.
18. van den Bos R, Arends L, Kockaert M, et al. Endovenous therapies of lower extremity varicosities: a meta-analysis. J Vasc Surg 2009;49(1):230–9.
19. Lurie F, Creton D, Eklof B, et al. Prospective randomised study of EndoVenous radiofrequency obliteration (closure) versus Ligation and VEin Stripping (EVOLVeS): two-year follow-up. Eur J Vasc Endovasc Surg 2005;29(1):67–73.
20. Darwood RJ, Theivacumar N, Dellagrammaticas D, et al. Randomized clinical trial comparing endovenous laser ablation with surgery for the treatment of primary great saphenous varicose veins. Br J Surg 2008;95(3):294–301.
21. Rasmussen LH, Lawaetz M, Bjoern L, et al. Randomized clinical trial comparing endovenous laser ablation, radiofrequency ablation, foam sclerotherapy and surgical stripping for great saphenous varicose veins. Br J Surg 2011;98(8): 1079–87.
22. Almeida JI, Javier JJ, Mackay E, et al. First human use of cyanoacrylate adhesive for treatment of saphenous vein incompetence. J Vasc Surg Venous Lymphat Disord 2013;1(2):174–80.
23. Proebstle TM, Alm J, Dimitri S, et al. The European multicenter cohort study on cyanoacrylate embolization of refluxing great saphenous veins. J Vasc Surg Venous Lymphat Disord 2015;3(1):2–7.
24. Holewijn S, van Eekeren RRJP, Vahl A, et al. Two-year results of a multicenter randomized controlled trial comparing Mechanochemical endovenous Ablation to RADiOfrequeNcy Ablation in the treatment of primary great saphenous vein incompetence (MARADONA trial). J Vasc Surg Venous Lymphat Disord 2019; 7(3):364–74.
25. Neglén P, Raju S. Intravascular ultrasound scan evaluation of the obstructed vein. J Vasc Surg 2002;35(4):694–700.

Perioperative Respiratory Concerns in the Surgical Patient

Gayle B. Bodner, MMS, PA-C[a,b,*]

KEYWORDS

- Preoperative optimization • Postoperative pulmonary complications
- Chronic lung disease • Obstructive sleep apnea

KEY POINTS

- Postoperative pulmonary complications are costly and common and contribute to significant morbidity and mortality.
- It is important to have a high suspicion in surgical patient case planning.
- Preoperative assessment is ideal for risk stratification, medical optimization, and planning for postoperative monitoring and management.
- There are many independent risk factors for postoperative pulmonary complications; characteristics of the surgery are often a greater predictor than patient related factors.
- Several tools exist to help clinicians identify risk.

INTRODUCTION

Respiratory concerns in the perioperative setting are common and costly and impact patient morbidity and mortality. Predictors of pulmonary complications are multifaceted, including components of time, acuity, patient-specific risk factors, and often, most important, characteristics of the surgery. These concerns can arise acutely during the perioperative course in patients with or without chronic comorbidities. A review of the entire scope of respiratory concerns in the perioperative setting is not the intention of this article. This review addresses salient considerations for the adult surgical patient.

Although cardiovascular complications are well-defined and often in the forefront of risk assessment, postoperative pulmonary complications (PPC) are more costly and common.[1] They can also be associated with increased length of stay and increased morbidity and mortality.[2] The incidence of PPC varies widely in the literature, ranging from 3% to 40%,[3,4] depending on how the complication was defined as well as the

[a] Department of Anesthesiology, Wake Forest School of Medicine, Winston Salem, NC, USA;
[b] Department of PA Studies, Wake Forest School of Medicine, Winston Salem, NC, USA
* Medical Center Boulevard, Winston Salem, NC 27127.
E-mail address: gbodner@wakehealth.edu

Physician Assist Clin 6 (2021) 331–342
https://doi.org/10.1016/j.cpha.2020.11.009
2405-7991/21/© 2020 Elsevier Inc. All rights reserved.
physicianassistant.theclinics.com

surgical population. These included definitions such as respiratory infections, exacerbation of existing pulmonary disease, hypoxemia, and the need for invasive or noninvasive mechanical ventilation. Other definitions have been more specific and include laryngospasm, bronchospasm, aspiration, airway obstruction, pulmonary barotrauma, pneumothorax, pulmonary edema, pleural effusion, and pulmonary embolism. Based on the wide range of definitions, the interpretation of PPC in individual patient groups can be challenging. Additionally, there has been some criticism of the databases used for risk prediction, because they have not all been sufficiently heterogeneous with respect to sex, race, or geographic area.

PREOPERATIVE IDENTIFICATION

The preoperative setting is ideal to identify patients at higher risk for PPC. Predicting patients who are at higher risk gives an opportunity to optimize acute or chronic medical conditions and may even include using a delay in surgery when appropriate. Identification also allows for advance surgical and anesthetic planning to minimize risk when possible. With that, lies potential for impact on health care system resources and costs. Finally, identification allows for patient education and enriches the discussion of informed consent.

A preoperative evaluation should include a thorough history and physical examination. A review of the past medical history for chronic diseases and current management with particular emphasis on smoking history, presence of congestive heart failure (CHF), any chronic lung disease, previous pulmonary complications, and the presence or risk of obstructive sleep apnea (OSA) is important. In these patients, one should ask about any oxygen requirements, previous hospitalization for their chronic condition, and if they had prior perioperative exacerbation of their disease.

A patient's ability to complete activities of daily living as well as exercise can be helpful in uncovering underlying cardiac or pulmonary disease. This process can include asking about self-care, household chores, yard work, or the ability to climb stairs as a gauge for their cardiopulmonary status. Important symptoms include dyspnea, chest discomfort or near-syncope that could indicate preexisting pulmonary disease such as chronic obstructive pulmonary disease (COPD) or cardiac disease such as CHF, cardiac ischemia, structural heart disease, or arrhythmias. Identification and assessment of any fever, wheezing, worsening cough, sputum, dyspnea, or snoring is essential. Symptoms of orthopnea, paroxysmal nocturnal dyspnea, snoring, and weight gain can be beneficial in identifying CHF or OSA.

Physical examination can reveal resting hypoxia and identify difficult airway markers, such as poor cervical range of motion, large tongue, and/or a high Mallampati score. The Mallampati classification is based on what structures are visible at eye level with the patient holding the head in a neutral position, opening the mouth widely, and protruding the tongue without phonation. Class III (only the soft palate and base of the uvula are visible) and class IV (uvula and soft palate are not visible) correlate with a potential for difficult intubation.

At minimum, a focused examination of the lungs and heart can identify wheezing, decreased breath sounds, rhonchi, prolonged expiration, and other markers of acute or chronic pulmonary or cardiac disease. Cardiac examination findings of an elevated jugular venous pressure, murmurs, S3 or S4, loud P2, heaves, and abdominal or lower extremity edema can raise concern for heart failure or other structural heart disease.

Documentation of these factors aids the perioperative care team in knowing the patient's baseline signs and symptoms and can assist in optimal perioperative management. For patients with respiratory concerns, understanding the patient's history and physical examination can direct decisions about intubation and choices of anesthetic. It also helps to inform postoperative respiratory support and pain management. For many patients, it is an opportunity to arrange diagnostic studies to address possibilities raised during the evaluation as well as to arrange for specialist consultation.

RISK FACTORS FOR POSTOPERATIVE PULMONARY COMPLICATIONS

To begin looking at risk factors, a patient's age can be an independent risk factor. The majority of studies indicate risk increases at age 60 and older[5,6] with a more recent study showing risk at an age of more than 50 years.[7] The greatest risk is noted with patients more than 80 years of age.[7,8] Another independent risk factor is American Society of Anesthesiologists (ASA) class which is noted in **Table 1**. An ASA class II or more is a risk factor, with risk increasing at higher ASA levels.[3,5,8,9] Functional dependence,[3,5,8] defined as partial or total dependence for activities of daily living is a risk factor. Smoking, which is prevalent in the surgical patient population is another risk factor.[7,8] More recent investigations indicate that a preoperative supine oxygen saturation of 90% or less is a strong predictor.[7] Independent risk factors for PPC are listed in **Table 2**.

COPD is also an independent risk factor. Analyzing data from the American College of Surgeons National Surgical Quality Improvement Program (NSQIP) database, Gupta and colleagues[10] found that patients with COPD had an overall mortality rate of 6.7% compared with 1.4% without the disease. They also noted that COPD was independently associated with postoperative pneumonia, respiratory failure, myocardial infarction, sepsis, renal failure requiring dialysis, and wound dehiscence after controlling for more than 50 comorbidities and type of surgery.

Of all the risk factors, however, surgery-related risk factors were the greatest predictors of PPC,[2,5,7,8] even in healthy patients. The type of surgery is a major predictor. Open aortic surgeries confer the greatest risk of complications,[5] followed by thoracic, abdominal, neurosurgery, head and neck, and vascular surgeries. When looking at major abdominal surgeries, Yang and colleagues[8] found the greatest risk factor for PPCs was in patients who underwent esophagectomy, noting a more than 5 times higher risk of PPC. Surgical location with proximity to the diaphragm has frequently been used to evaluate risk by type of surgery.

Prolonged surgery also is an independent risk factor, with surgeries longer than 2 to 4 hours[6,7,9] carrying an increased risk. Another surgery-related risk factor is the acuity of the surgical condition. Emergency surgery confers a much higher incidence of PPC compared with nonemergent surgeries.[6,7,9]

In summary, there are multiple independent risk factors for PPC. Surgery-related risk factors confer the greatest risk, even in a healthy patient, with a particular emphasis on the type of surgery. Thoracic and upper abdominal procedures have been well-documented to increase risk as well as a duration of more than 2 to 4 hours and emergency surgeries.

ANESTHESIA-RELATED FACTORS

Residual effects of anesthetics and narcotics in conjunction with decreased pulmonary capacity owing to pain and potential diaphragmatic dysfunction can lead to regional atelectasis[11] and hypoxemia. A patient may have a limited ability to clear respiratory secretions, which can worsen hypoxemia and can increase the risk of respiratory infections. Large volumes of fluid or blood products administered in the perioperative period can also contribute to adverse pulmonary complications. One uncommon complication to note is transfusion-related lung injury, because it carries a

Table 1		
ASA physical status classification system		
ASA PS Classification	**Definition**	**Examples, Including, But Not Limited to:**
ASA I	A normal healthy patient	Healthy, nonsmoking, no or minimal alcohol use
ASA II	A patient with mild systemic disease	Mild diseases only without substantive functional limitations. Examples include (but not limited to): current smoker, social alcohol drinker, pregnancy, obesity (30 < BMI < 40), well-controlled DM/HTN, mild lung disease
ASA III	A patient with severe systemic disease	Substantive functional limitations. One or more moderate to severe diseases. Examples include (but not limited to): poorly controlled DM or HTN, COPD, morbid obesity (BMI ≥40), active hepatitis, alcohol dependence or abuse, implanted pacemaker, moderate reduction of ejection fraction, ESRD undergoing regularly scheduled dialysis, premature infant PCA <60 wk, history (>3 mo) of MI, CVA, TIA, or CAD/stents.
ASA IV	A patient with severe systemic disease that is a constant threat to life	Examples include (but not limited to): recent (<3 mo) MI, CVA, TIA, or CAD/stents, ongoing cardiac ischemia or severe valve dysfunction, severe reduction of ejection fraction, sepsis, DIC, ARD, or ESRD not undergoing regularly scheduled dialysis
ASA V	A moribund patient who is not expected to survive without the operation	Examples include (but not limited to): ruptured abdominal/thoracic aneurysm, massive trauma, intracranial bleed with mass effect, ischemic bowel in the face of significant cardiac pathology or multiple organ/system dysfunction
ASA VI	A declared brain-dead patient whose organs are being removed for donor purposes	

Abbreviations: ARD, acute respiratory disease; BMI, body mass index; CAD, coronary artery disease; CVA, cerebrovascular accident; DIC, disseminated intravascular coagulation; DM, diabetes mellitus; ESRD, end-stage renal disease; HTN, hypertension; MI, myocardial infarction; PCA, patient-controlled analgesia; TIA, transient ischemic attack.

*The addition of "E" denotes Emergency surgery: (An emergency is defined as existing when delay in treatment of the patient would lead to a significant increase in the threat to life or body part).

American Society of Anesthesiologists. Developed By: ASA House of Delegates/Executive Committee. Last Amended: October 23, 2019. http://asahq.org/resources/clinical-information/asa-physical-status-classification-system.

Table 2 Risk factors for PPCs	
Patient Related	**Procedure Related**
Age >50 or >60 y	Emergency surgery
ASA > II	Prolonged surgery
CHF or pulmonary hypertension	General anesthesia
Functional dependence	Surgical site
COPD	Aortic aneurysm repair
Impaired sensorium	Head and neck surgery
Albumin <3.5	Thoracic surgery
OSA	Abdominal surgery
Preoperative SpO$_2$ <90	Vascular surgery
Respiratory infection in last month	Neurosurgery
Preoperative anemia (hemoglobin <10)	
Smoking	

Data from Qaseem et al. Annals of Internal Medicine 144:575-580.and Mazo et al. Anesthesiology 2014; 121:219-231.

significant risk of mortality. The actual or highly suspected transfusion-related lung injury incidence is low, approximately 1.4% in noncardiac surgery.[12]

In a systematic review and meta-analysis by Uhlig and colleagues,[13] patients undergoing general anesthesia for cardiac surgery were found to have a lower mortality and lower incidence of PPC with volatile (inhaled) anesthetics compared with total intravenous anesthesia. This was felt to be due to properties of these agents, which include coronary vasodilation as well as bronchodilation. In that study, however, there was no decreased mortality benefit or decrease in PPC noted in patients undergoing noncardiac surgery.[13]

For patients with COPD, there can be a concern for delayed extubation and prolonged ventilator support with the use of general anesthesia. Ultimately, the choice of anesthesia is determined by the anesthesia team, but communication among the teams may include a discussion of regional anesthesia. Regional anesthesia can include epidural or spinal anesthesia with or without peripheral nerve blocks. In a retrospective, propensity-matched cohort study of NSQIP database-defined patients with severe COPD, the use of spinal anesthesia was associated with lower incidences of pneumonia, prolonged ventilator dependence, unplanned postoperative intubation, and composite morbidity.[14] However, this benefit decreased in the sickest of the patients (those with baseline dyspnea at rest and/or ASA class IV) and there was no mortality benefit. In that study, severe COPD was characterized clinically as functional disability from COPD, previous hospitalization for COPD, chronic bronchodilator therapy requirement, or a forced expiratory volume in 1 second that is less than 75% of predicted value on pulmonary function testing. Additionally, pain control with a postoperative epidural can improve pulmonary function, decrease the risk of infection, and improve the 30-day mortality in patients with COPD.[14,15]

In patients with a known or predicted difficult airway, there is concern for failure to maintain the airway. Potential adverse complications related to difficult airway include death, brain injury, cardiopulmonary arrest, unnecessary surgical airway, airway trauma, and damage to the teeth.[16]

RISK PREDICTION

Risk prediction tools exist that include incorporate both patient- and surgical-related risk factors. Data from the American College of Surgeons NSQIP database was used in 2 risk calculators, the NSQIP Respiratory Failure Risk Tool, which predicts development of respiratory failure, and the NSQIP Pneumonia Risk Tool, which predicts the risk of postoperative pneumonia, both within 30 days of surgery.[2,4] Postoperative respiratory failure is defined as failure to wean from mechanical ventilation within 48 hours of surgery or unplanned intubation/reintubation postoperatively.

More than 200,000 patients were used for tool development, and a similar but different cohort was used for validation. These cohorts included a diversity of surgeries, both emergent and nonemergent. The tools address postoperative respiratory failure and pneumonia, respectively, but do not discriminate other types of PPC.

Both tools include ASA class, type of surgery, and functional status. The respiratory failure risk tool also includes emergency surgery, and the pneumonia risk tool includes smoking, patient age, and the presence of COPD. These tools are easy to use and available at https://www.mdcalc.com/gupta-postoperative-respiratory-failure-risk and https://www.mdcalc.com/gupta-postoperative-pneumonia-risk.

A prospective, observational, multicenter European study included patients undergoing emergent and nonemergent surgery with general, combined, or regional anesthesia techniques. This study was used to validate the Assess Respiratory Risk in Surgical Patients in Catalonia Tool (ARISCAT).[9,17] The ARISCAT score[9] uses 7 patient- and surgical-related risk factors (surgical site, preoperative oxygen saturation, duration of surgery, recent pulmonary infection, age, anemia, and emergency status) to stratify risk into 3 categories (low, intermediate, and high). Access to this tool is available at https://www.mdcalc.com/ariscat-score-postoperative-pulmonary-complications#evidence.

The ARISCAT score can be a helpful tool; however, a limitation has been noted to include applicability to US patients owing to evaluation differences found in European patient groups.

PREOPERATIVE TESTING

Specific, indicated testing is recommended in the preoperative setting; however, routine preoperative testing of every patient has fallen out of favor. Routine testing of patients without an indication can yield abnormal results that have the potential for unnecessary delays, patient anxiety, and inappropriate interventions. In circumstances where the abnormal result does not affect the patient's anesthetic or surgical course, patient risk and financial cost are often not justified. Using information from the patient history and physical examination will help to guide and select appropriate testing. Indicated testing provides information that may change patient management, thereby supporting justification for risk and cost.

In a patient with suspected new or worsening cardiac or pulmonary disease, a chest radiograph can be helpful, as well as in the evaluation of suspected pulmonary infection. Chest radiographs do not add value in a stable patient. Pulmonary function testing can be used for patients who are suspected of asthma or COPD, but not yet diagnosed. They are also commonly used to determine pulmonary capacity before lung resection surgery.

Arterial blood gases can be beneficial in patients with baseline CO_2 retention and/ or oxygen dependence, but use should take into account other factors such as postoperative disposition and surgery related factors. An electrocardiogram can be useful to evaluate other causes of cardiopulmonary symptoms and assess for right heart strain. Echocardiography is indicated if heart failure is suspected as a cause of dyspnea or to characterize the severity of existing cardiopulmonary disease. Right heart catheterization is invasive and expensive and used primarily to delineate the severity of pulmonary hypertension.

DECREASING RISK

Minimally invasive surgical techniques may minimize some PPC[11] and can be considered, if surgically appropriate, as well as anesthetic strategies. When a change to the surgical or anesthetic approach is not reasonable or feasible, focused optimization of medical conditions can be helpful and inform the patient discussion.

Preoperatively, patients with underlying respiratory disease should be optimized if possible. Respiratory tract infections should be addressed, treated, and, in most cases, consideration should be made to postpone elective surgery. Postponement is often for 4 to 8 weeks, but can vary depending on severity.

Additionally, the preoperative setting is ideal for addressing smoking cessation. Smoking cessation is advised, although optimal timing varies in the literature from 1 to 2 months.[6,8,18] A systematic review and meta-analysis by Grønkjoer and colleagues[18] noted that tobacco use preoperatively correlated with increased rates of postoperative morbidity, infection, prolonged wound healing, neurologic complications, intensive care unit admissions, and PPCs.

A smoking cessation strategy has been shown to decrease postoperative complications and should be implemented as early as possible.[19] Patients can receive counseling and support, be directed to nicotine replacement, and consideration of medical therapy such as bupropion or varenicline.

CHRONIC LUNG DISEASE

Asthma that is well-controlled has not been found to be a risk for intraoperative or postoperative complications. Patients who have poor control, particularly those with active wheezing at the time of induction, are at a higher risk of complications.[20] Elective surgery should not be performed in patients with active bronchospasm. The surgery should be delayed until the cause and symptoms can be treated to the point where the patient is at or as near as possible to their baseline status.[20]

Patients with asthma should be advised to avoid known environmental triggers in the days leading up to surgery and report changes in symptoms. Prophylactic short-acting bronchodilator therapy, via metered dose inhaler or nebulizer, is felt to be beneficial.[20] In patients with poorly controlled asthma, short courses of preoperative corticosteroids can be considered without the risk of postoperative infections[20] or significant adrenal suppression. Although the risk of severe perioperative bronchospasm is relatively low in asthmatic patients, it can be life threatening. Therefore, a careful preoperative assessment, optimal timing of the surgery, anesthetic planning, and careful postoperative monitoring are important. Stable patients should be encouraged to continue their usual asthma treatment regimen.

COPD is common in the surgical patient population.[10] When compared with similar patients without the diagnosis, patients with COPD have longer average operative times and spend 4 times as long recovering in the hospital.[10,21] As noted elsewhere in this article, it is an independent risk factor for PPC. In a retrospective study of 405 patients with COPD, Kim and colleagues[21] found that PPC occurred in 29% of patients and the greatest risks were in those undergoing thoracic and upper abdominal surgery. Additionally, pneumonia was the most common PPC, followed by pleural effusion and atelectasis.

There are few data suggesting alternative management of the preoperative patient with COPD. Surgical delay should be considered for any patient who is having an exacerbation until they resume or are near their baseline function. Existing treatment includes inhaled beta agonists, anticholinergics, systemic or inhaled corticosteroids, and supplemental oxygen, and these modalities should be continued, including on the day of surgery. In asthma or COPD, in an effort to decrease PPC, short courses of oral or intravenous corticosteroids have been used, although there is mixed evidence to support their use.[20,22,23] Patients should be encouraged to be current on vaccinations, including pneumococcal, if appropriate.

Other considerations include nutritional optimization[11] because malnutrition and hypoalbuminemia increase the risk of PPC.[6] If time and resources are available, pulmonary prehabilitation (exercise training, secretion clearance techniques, and incentive spirometry) can be beneficial for patients with poor capacity.

Restrictive lung disease or chronic disease that may predispose to lung restriction, such as chest wall deformity and neuromuscular disease are not as well-studied. Surgical teams may consider patients with severe limitations to have an increased risk of PPC.[6]

SLEEP APNEA

Sleep apnea can include central sleep apnea, obesity hypoventilation syndrome, and OSA. This section addresses OSA, but many concepts apply to all 3 conditions. Patients with severe apnea are at risk for severe pulmonary hypertension, which carries its own perioperative risks.

Sleep-disordered breathing can have different causes and is often not diagnosed by the time of surgery.[24] Advanced age and obesity are often contributing factors in the surgical population. Patients with OSA tend to have a more narrow and collapsible pharyngeal airway owing to a larger tongue, soft palate, and/or peripharyngeal fat. OSA is important to recognize because it can impact the ability to mask ventilate the patient as well as hinder direct laryngoscopy or fiber optic visualization of the airway and endotracheal intubation. In addition to being at higher risk for difficult intubation or reintubation, patients with OSA are at risk for hypercapnia, oxygen desaturation,[25] airway obstruction, pneumonia, and a longer hospitalization.[26] Additionally, these patients are more sensitive to respiratory depression with the administration of opioids, sedatives, and inhaled anesthetics.[27] When compared with similar patients without the diagnosis, patients with OSA are at a higher risk for PPC.[24]

Memtsoudis and colleagues[25] sampled inpatient data for lower extremity joint arthroplasty and open abdominal surgeries. They found that OSA increased the odds ratio by 5-fold for perioperative intubation and mechanical ventilation after orthopedic surgery and twice the odds for open abdominal surgery patients when compared with matched controls without OSA.

Expert consensus guidelines recommend screening for OSA,[24] even though there has not been an abundance of evidence that the use of preoperative screening tools for OSA to decrease patient complications. There is limited evidence to support canceling or delaying a surgery to pursue polysomnography and positive airway pressure (PAP) therapy, unless there is evidence of systemic disease such as severe pulmonary hypotension or hypoventilation.[24] In those cases, referral for cardiopulmonary optimization should be strongly considered. One tool to screen for OSA is STOP-Bang[28] and can be found at https://www.mdcalc.com/stop-bang-score-obstructive-sleep-apnea.

Preoperatively, a discussion should include the risks associated with OSA. In patients with OSA, PAP therapy may help to decrease PPC based on observational data.[27] Therefore, if appropriate, patients should use their device postoperatively and throughout their hospitalization. Including documentation of their polysomnography and PAP settings can help to inform the type of anesthesia, analgesia regimens, and postoperative monitoring.

PULMONARY HYPERTENSION

Pulmonary hypertension can be a heterogeneous disease process that poses a significant risk for patients requiring surgery. Primary considerations are hypoxia and volume shifts that exacerbate the underlying disease and lead to right heart failure. In this population, postoperative complications include coronary ischemia, persistent hypoxia, pulmonary embolism, and right ventricular failure leading to postoperative respiratory failure and/or death.[29]

Preoperatively, the main goal is to identify their presence if there is clinical suspicion by echocardiographic estimation of the pulmonary artery pressure. In patients with confirmed disease, case planning should include a pulmonary hypertension specialist,[30] as well as the surgeon and anesthesiologist. Postoperatively, the patient's volume status should be assessed diligently to avoid cardiovascular collapse and hypoxemia should be minimized.

For any patient with a very high risk of PPC (severe cases of COPD, OSA, or pulmonary hypertension), the risk must be weighed against the potential benefit of the surgery. There is no specific severity of pulmonary disease that has been recognized as an absolute contraindication to surgery.

VENOUS THROMBOEMBOLISM

Venous thromboembolism is a known complication of surgical procedures. Risk factors for postoperative venous thromboembolism include advanced age, certain types of surgery (eg, lower extremity, abdominal, spine), the presence of malignancy, the presence of a central venous catheter, complete or prolonged immobility, certain thrombophilias, previous venous thromboembolism, CHF, chronic pulmonary disease, pregnancy, and some medications, such as hormonal therapy.

A calculator from the American College of Surgeons NSQIP uses 20 predictors in addition to the planned procedure to predict outcomes within 30 days of surgery. This calculator provides estimates of many complications. The output for serious complications encompasses many dire pulmonary and cardiac events, including pulmonary embolus. Venous thromboembolism is also calculated separately with other events. Entering the most complete patient data will improve risk estimates; however, clinicians can still run the estimate when some patient information is not known. That calculator is located at https://riskcalculator.facs.org/RiskCalculator/.

Patients can present with dyspnea, tachycardia, acute hypoxia, hemoptysis, chest pain, unilateral lower extremity edema, or pain. Because other postoperative considerations can lead to these signs and symptoms, clinical suspicion is vital.

POSTOPERATIVE CARE

In the abdominal surgery population, PPC can develop over a longer period of time with a median of 4 to 6 days.[8] Recognizing a higher risk patient gives an opportunity to optimize the patient's pulmonary function while addressing pain control and early ambulation.[6] Chest physiotherapy, deep breathing exercises, and incentive spirometry have proven benefits with minimal adverse effects and can contribute to improved respiratory outcomes in high-risk patients. If the patient cannot participate, consider noninvasive positive pressure ventilation if appropriate.[11]

Patients at increased perioperative risk from OSA should be extubated while awake unless there is a medical or surgical contraindication. Extubation and recovery should be carried out in the lateral, semi-upright, or other nonsupine positions when possible.[27]

Oximetry is recommended for patients at high risk of hypoxemia. In patients who remain on a ventilator, consider protocols to minimize ventilator-associated pneumonia including semi-upright bed positioning and a plan for weaning.

Enhanced recovery after surgery is an evidence-based effort to provide integrated perioperative care to surgical patients to improve patient outcomes. One common component of enhanced recovery after surgery includes multimodal pain management.[15] This practice can include ice/heat, transcutaneous electrical nerve stimulation, acetaminophen, nonsteroidal anti-inflammatory drugs, gabapentinoids, regional analgesia, and other agents to minimize the use of opiates, which are associated with increased apneic events, hypoxia, and hypercarbia. Sedatives, such as benzodiazepines or barbiturates can also increase these risks. Regional anesthesia techniques with potential opioid-sparing effects may be used when safe and appropriate; postoperative epidural analgesia may decrease respiratory muscle dysfunction and hypoventilation associated with pain.[11] Additionally, appropriate pain management allows for patient mobilization for improved clearance of respiratory secretions.

Nasogastric tube placement is generally not recommended postoperatively, except in cases of nausea and vomiting, symptomatic abdominal distension, or poor oral intake. When used selectively, it may decrease the incidence of PPC after elective abdominal surgery.[11]

For patients with OSA treated with PAP therapy, it should be resumed postoperatively as soon as feasible. Empiric PAP should be considered postoperatively in patients with OSA who were not using it preoperatively, particularly when there are periods of hypoxemia, hypoventilation, or observed apnea.

SUMMARY

Perioperative pulmonary complications are common, costly, and associated with high morbidity and mortality, and the predictors are largely based on aspects of the surgery itself as well as some clinical indicators. Surgical care teams should use a multipronged approach to minimize PPC, which includes perioperative evaluation and optimization, informed patient discussion about risk, exploration of potential surgical and anesthetic alternatives, and the use of postoperative interventions that decrease risk. A high suspicion of PPC is vital in preoperative discussion, case planning, and postoperative management.

CLINICS CARE POINTS

- In a patient with poor functional capacity, their ability to complete activities in the absence of cardiopulmonary symptoms can be helpful as a measure of exercise. Consider household chores, yard work, or the ability to climb stairs as examples.
- When respiratory concerns arise, coordination with the surgical and anesthesia teams is often overlooked. Open lines of communication can improve efficiency, patient experience and when case planning is adjusted accordingly, potential for better patient outcomes.

DISCLOSURE

The author has nothing to disclose.

REFERENCES

1. Dimick JB, Chen SL, Taheri PA, et al. Hospital costs associated with surgical complications: a report from the private-sector National Surgical Quality Improvement Program. J Am Coll Surg 2004;199(4):531–7.
2. Gupta H, Gupta PK, Schuller D, et al. Development and validation of a risk calculator for predicting postoperative pneumonia. Mayo Clin Proc 2013;88:1241–9.
3. Bapoje SR, Whitaker JF, Schulz T, et al. Preoperative evaluation of the patient with pulmonary disease. Chest 2007;132(5):1637–45.
4. Gupta H, Gupta PK, Fang X, et al. Development and validation of a risk calculator predicting postoperative respiratory failure. Chest 2011;140(5):1207–15.
5. Smetana GW, Lawrence VA, Cornell JE, et al. Preoperative pulmonary risk stratification for noncardiothoracic surgery: systematic review for the American College of Physicians. Ann Intern Med 2006;144(8):581–95.
6. Qaseem A, Snow V, Fitterman N, et al. Risk assessment for and strategies to reduce perioperative pulmonary complications for patients undergoing noncardiothoracic surgery: a guideline from the American College of Physicians. Ann Intern Med 2006;144:575–80.
7. Canet J, Gallart L, Gomar C, et al, ARISCAT Group. Prediction of postoperative pulmonary complications in a population-based surgical cohort. Anesthesiology 2010;113(6):1338–50.
8. Yang CK, Teng A, Lee DY, et al. Pulmonary complications after major abdominal surgery: National Surgical Quality Improvement Program analysis. J Surg Res 2015;198(2):441–9.
9. Mazo V, Sabaté S, Canet J, et al. Prospective external validation of a predictive score for postoperative pulmonary complications. Anesthesiology 2014;121: 219–31.
10. Gupta H, Ramanan B, Gupta PK, et al. Impact of COPD on postoperative outcomes: results from a national database. Chest 2013;143(6):1599–606.
11. Lawrence VA, Cornell JE, Smetana GW. Strategies to reduce postoperative pulmonary complications after noncardiothoracic surgery: systematic review for the American College of Physicians. Ann Intern Med 2006;144(8):596–608.
12. Clifford L, Jia Q, Subramanian A, et al. Characterizing the epidemiology of postoperative transfusion-related acute lung injury. Anesthesiology 2015;122(1): 12–20.
13. Uhlig C, Bluth T, Schwarz K, et al. Effects of volatile anesthetics on mortality and postoperative pulmonary and other complications in patients undergoing surgery: a systematic review and meta-analysis. Anesthesiology 2016;124(6): 1230–45.
14. Hausman MS Jr, Jewell ES, Engoren M. Regional versus general anesthesia in surgical patients with chronic obstructive pulmonary disease: does avoiding general anesthesia reduce the risk of postoperative complications? Anesth Analg 2015;120(6):1405–12.
15. Wick EC, Grant MC, Wu CL. Postoperative multimodal analgesia pain management with nonopioid analgesics and techniques: a review. JAMA Surg 2017; 152(7):691–7.
16. Practice guidelines for management of the difficult airway: an updated report by the American Society of Anesthesiologists task force on management of the difficult airway. Anesthesiology 2013;118:251–70.
17. Russotto B, Sabaté S, Canet J, PERISCOPE Group of the European Society of Anaesthesiology (ESA) Clinical Trial Network. Development of a prediction model

for postoperative pneumonia: a multicentre prospective observational study. Eur J Anaesthesiol 2019;36:93–104.

18. Grønkjoer M, Eliasen M, Skov-Ettrup LS, et al. Preoperative smoking status and postoperative complications: a systematic review and meta-analysis. Ann Surg 2014;259(1):52–71.

19. Mills E, Eyawo O, Lockhart I, et al. Smoking cessation reduces postoperative complications: a systematic review and meta-analysis. Am J Med 2011;124(2): 144–54.

20. Woods BD, Sladen RN. Perioperative considerations for the patient with asthma and bronchospasm. Br Anaesth 2009;103(suppl 1):i57–65.

21. Kim HJ, Lee J, Park YS, et al. Impact of GOLD groups of chronic pulmonary obstructive disease on surgical complications. Int J Chron Obstruct Pulmon Dis 2016;11:281–7.

22. Lee HW, Lee JK, Oh SH, et al. Effect of perioperative systemic steroid treatment on patients with obstructive lung disease undergoing elective abdominal surgery. Clin Respir J 2018;12(1):227–33.

23. Arbid SA, El-Khoury H, Jamali F, et al. Association of preoperative systemic corticosteroid therapy with surgical outcomes in chronic obstructive pulmonary disease patients. Ann Thorac Med 2019;14(2):141–7.

24. Chung F, Memtsoudis SG, Ramachandran SK, et al. Society of Anesthesia and Sleep Medicine Guidelines on Preoperative Screening and Assessment of Adult Patients With Obstructive Sleep Apnea. Anesth Analg 2016;123(2):452–73.

25. Memtsoudis S, Liu SS, Ma Y, et al. Perioperative pulmonary outcomes in patients with sleep apnea after noncardiac surgery. Anesth Analg 2011;112(1):113–21.

26. Wijeysundera DN, Sweitzer BJ. Preoperative evaluation. In: Miller RD, editor. Miller's anesthesia. 8th edition. Philadelphia: Elsevier Inc; 2015. p. 1085–155.e7.

27. Practice Guidelines for the Perioperative Management of Patients with Obstructive Sleep Apnea An Updated Report by the American Society of Anesthesiologists Task Force on Perioperative Management of Patients with Obstructive Sleep Apnea. Anesthesiology 2014;120(2):268–86.

28. Chung F, Yang Y, Liao P. Predictive performance of the STOP-Bang score for identifying obstructive sleep apnea in obese patients. Obes Surg 2013;23(12): 2050–7.

29. Ramakrishna G, Sprung J, Ravi BS, et al. Impact of pulmonary hypertension on the outcomes of noncardiac surgery: predictors of perioperative morbidity and mortality. J Am Coll Cardiol 2005;45(10):1691–9.

30. Fleisher LA, Fleischmann KE, Auerbach AD, et al. American College of Cardiology; American Heart Association. 2014 ACC/AHA guideline on perioperative cardiovascular evaluation and management of patients undergoing noncardiac surgery: a report of the American College of Cardiology/American Heart Association Task Force on Practice Guidelines. J Am Coll Cardiol 2014;64(22):e77–137.

Gender-Affirming Genitourinary Surgery

Kayla McLaughlin, PA-C[a],*, Melissa M. Poh, MD[a], Amanda C. Chi, MD[b],
Holly H. Kim, MD[c], Polina Reyblat, MD[b]

KEYWORDS

- Gender Dysphoria • Transgender • Vaginoplasty • Phalloplasty • Neovagina
- Neourethra • Nonbinary • Gender Diverse

KEY POINTS

- An affirmative, multidisciplinary team including medical and mental health specialists should be used throughout the surgical process.
- The penile-inversion approach to vaginoplasty consists of creation and lining of the vaginal canal (neovagina), shortening and repositioning of the urethra, construction of the neoclitoris, and rearrangement of local tissues to form the vulvar anatomy.
- Several degrees of surgical transition exist for transmen: hysterectomy with or without salpingo-oophorectomy; removal of the vaginal canal; creation of male external genitalia with or without lengthening of the urethra; placement of testicular and/or penile prosthesis.
- Binary transition (male to female or female to male) is not a requirement for surgery; therefore, individual goals of surgical transition should be carefully discussed between the patient and the multidisciplinary team, and in accordance with the World Professional Association for Transgender Health (WPATH) standards of care.

 Video content accompanies this article at http://www.physicianassistant. theclinics.com.

INTRODUCTION

Recent years have seen a significant increase in health care initiatives for transgender and gender variant persons caused by better awareness of gender dysphoria both in society and among the medical community. In 2014, Section 1557 of the Affordable Care Act prohibited insurance coverage discrimination based on gender identity and Medicare began coverage of gender-affirming surgeries.[1] As a result, many

[a] Department of Plastic Surgery, Kaiser Permanente, 6041 Cadillac Avenue, Los Angeles, CA 90034, USA; [b] Department of Urology, Kaiser Permanente, 6041 Cadillac Avenue, Los Angeles, CA 90034, USA; [c] Transition Pathways Clinic, Kaiser Permanente, 6041 Cadillac Avenue, Los Angeles, CA 90034, USA
* Corresponding author.
E-mail address: Kayla.c.mclaughlin@kp.org

Physician Assist Clin 6 (2021) 343–360
https://doi.org/10.1016/j.cpha.2020.11.010   physicianassistant.theclinics.com
2405-7991/21/© 2020 Elsevier Inc. All rights reserved.

state-sponsored and private insurance plans have broadened coverage to include transgender care.[2] Although many transgender people do not desire surgical transition, The US Trans Survey 2015, which includes almost 28,000 transgender and nonbinary participants, indicated that 42% of transgender men, 28% of transgender women, and 9% of gender nonbinary individuals had undergone at least 1 gender-affirming surgery.[3]

The increased demand for gender-inclusive surgical care has shown a need for health care provider education regarding both medical and surgical transition. More specifically, access to informed postoperative genitourinary care remains largely unavailable. This article provides a thorough overview of the preoperative assessment, surgical principles, and postoperative complications for gender-affirming surgery.

The penile-inversion vaginoplasty is the most common approach for vaginoplasty for male to female transition.[4] This surgery includes penile disassembly, bilateral orchiectomy, creation of a neovaginal canal between the bladder and rectum, labiaplasty, clitoroplasty, and urethroplasty.[5] Other techniques for vaginoplasty mostly differ in creation and lining of the neovaginal canal. Intestinal vaginoplasty involves use of a pedicled bowel transfer for neovaginal construction.

The main advantage of this technique is natural neovaginal lubrication and no need for preoperative genital hair removal. Drawbacks include the additional risk of abdominal surgery and malodorous discharge.[6] A peritoneal vaginoplasty is a surgical option for patients with inadequate penile or scrotal development and therefore insufficient skin to line the vaginal canal. Peritoneum can be harvested robotically or laparoscopically and added to the apex of the neovaginal canal.[7]

Surgical options for genitourinary female to male transition include simple or complex metoidioplasty and phalloplasty. Simple metoidioplasty involves release of the suspensory ligaments that tether the hormonally enlarged clitoris and use of local genital tissues such as labia minora to create a neophallus.[8] Complex metoidioplasty builds on the procedure described earlier with addition of urethral lengthening using local tissue and vaginectomy. Scrotoplasty may be combined with either a simple or a complex metoidioplasty. Phalloplasty refers to the creation of a neophallus from either a pedicled flap or free tissue transfer, such as a radial forearm free flap (RFFF) or a pedicled anterolateral thigh (ALT) flap.[9] Testicular and/or penile implants can be placed after full recovery from either gender-affirming procedure. However, penile implants are reserved for patients after phalloplasty because the neophallus in a metoidioplasty is insufficient to house an implant. Each of these procedures carries its own respective risks and complications that require consistent, well-informed follow-up.

GENERAL PRINCIPLES OF SURGICAL TREATMENT

As described by World Professional Association for Transgender Health (WPATH) standards of care (SOC), the goal of genitourinary surgical transition is to provide the affirmed genital morphology and alleviate gender dysphoria.[10] In the context of surgery, the goal is to create functional, sensate, aesthetically acceptable genitals and perineogenital anatomy that is congruent with the patient's gender identity.[11] Surgical consultation should include a thorough informed consent process with explanation of planned surgeries and associated risks and possible complications along with discussing the patient's surgical expectations. Preferably, transgender surgical care is provided under a multidisciplinary model with consistent communication between surgeons, primary care providers, mental health professionals, and endocrinologists. By the time of surgical consultation, patients should have met the guidelines for gender surgery defined by WPATH SOC, currently in its seventh edition with version 8 in development as of this writing. The process of meeting these guidelines can be arduous, and the surgical consultation can represent an important milestone in the patient's transition. The criteria for masculinizing metoidioplasty or phalloplasty and feminizing vaginoplasty are as follows:

1. Persistent, well-documented gender dysphoria
2. Capacity to make a fully informed decision and to give consent for treatment
3. Age of majority in a given country
4. If significant medical or mental health concerns are present, they must be well controlled
5. Twelve continuous months of hormone therapy as appropriate to the patient's gender goals (unless hormones are not indicated for the individual)
6. Twelve continuous months of living in a gender role that is congruent with the patient's gender identity

Requiring hormone therapy and living in the gender role congruent to the patient's gender identity allows the patient adequate time to experience a period of reversible endogenous hormone suppression and social transition before undergoing irreversible gonadectomy and complex surgery. The WPATH SOC are simply guidelines, and departures may be appropriate given an individual patient's anatomy, medical history, and surgical goals. Also note that binary transition is not a requirement for any gender-affirming surgery. For example, a transgender man may desire metoidioplasty, but forgo vaginectomy. Patients are required to obtain 2 mental health letters of support to establish that they have met the guidelines discussed earlier. These letters may be written by either primary care providers or mental health professionals. If any question as to whether surgery is indicated or judicious should arise, a discussion with the letter's author is encouraged, because the author may be more familiar with the patient's gender journey.[10]

General Preoperative Considerations

Preoperatively, medical comorbidities should be reasonably well controlled to minimize complications. Patients should be counseled on nicotine cessation and maintenance of a healthy body mass index (BMI) to modify risk of complications. Because of the use of skin/scrotal grafts and random skin flaps (penile shaft), nicotine cessation is imperative because of the compromise of dermal blood flow and increase in wound healing complications.[12]

Patients should abstain from all nicotine products for at least 2 months before surgery and at least 3 months postoperatively. It is useful for the patient to designate a caregiver for the surgery process, a consistent friend or family member who attends consultation and preoperative appointments so as to assist the patient during postoperative recovery. Mental health comorbidities can impair a patient's ability to adequately perform postoperative self-care and should be well controlled before surgery.

Fertility Preservation

Gender-affirming hormone therapy can negatively affect fertility to varying degrees and surgical gonadectomy results in infertility. WPATH SOC thus recommends discussing fertility and fertility preservation options before any gender-affirming treatment. Because WPATH recommends that patients receive at least 12 months of hormone therapy before gender-affirming genitourinary surgery, fertility preservation should be addressed before commencement of hormone supplementation or blockade. However, because patients' decisions toward, or access to, covered fertility preservation may have changed throughout their transition journeys, the option to preserve fertility should be addressed again before surgical gonadectomy.

Patients on testosterone

One of the goals of testosterone therapy is cessation of menses and suppression of ovulation, thereby affecting fertility while the patient is on treatment. However, fertility is not completely suppressed in all patients, and testosterone alone is not a reliable form of birth control if patients engage in sexual activity that can lead to pregnancy.[13] It is still unknown whether long-term use of testosterone therapy can permanently impair oocyte viability. There are reports of pregnancies in transgender men while actively on testosterone therapy and after more than 10 years of testosterone therapy.[14] Some patients undergoing gender-affirming metoidioplasty or phalloplasty may opt to retain their ovaries, and thus fertility could be retained. However, if oophorectomy is sought, patients should understand that infertility would be permanent and patients desiring future biological children should be counseled on oocyte and/or embryo cryopreservation. For oocyte retrieval, patients are referred to a fertility specialist for evaluation. Patients would need to suspend testosterone therapy for a period of time (4–6 weeks), followed by ovarian stimulation using medication and subsequent oocyte retrieval. Oocytes can be cryopreserved alone or fertilized to create embryos for implantation or cryopreservation.[15]

Patients on estrogen

Effects of estrogen therapy on the testes and sperm production is variable and dependent on the dose and length of treatment, so fertility preservation is best done before starting hormone therapy.[16] If estrogen has already been started, patients are advised to suspend estrogen and antiandrogens (eg, spironolactone) for 3 months to promote sperm viability. Patients can provide semen via ejaculation or can undergo testicular sperm extraction if needed. Sperm can be used for insemination or can be cryopreserved for future use.

TRANSFEMININE GENITOURINARY SURGERY PREOPERATIVE CONSIDERATIONS

The preoperative assessment for transfeminine patients should include a thorough history and physical examination, review of surgical options, and discussion of associated risks and possible complications. Several techniques for vaginoplasty are performed around the world, but the most common is the penile-inversion vaginoplasty. This procedure includes penectomy, orchiectomy, urethroplasty, labiaplasty, clitoroplasty, and creation of the neovaginal space between the bladder and rectum. Prostatectomy is not performed because of additional blood loss and risk of contributing to urinary incontinence. Patients should be educated on the need for continued prostate cancer screening. The neovaginal lining is derived from a superiorly based, inverted penile skin flap supplemented with a scrotal skin flap at the apex of the canal. Patients who have taken testosterone blockers since puberty may have limited genital development and therefore limited tissue to use in the reconstruction. In these cases, a skin graft from a separate donor site, such as lateral groin crease, may be necessary to supplement length. Any tissue that will be used to line the neovaginal canal and neovaginal introitus should undergo permanent hair removal, preferably through electrolysis. Laser hair removal may not be permanent and can result in collections of hair in the vaginal canal that can contribute to malodorous discharge and interfere with sexual activity and dilation. Patients who wish to avoid the added risk associated with neovaginal canal creation may elect to undergo shallow-depth vaginoplasty, also known as a zero-depth vaginoplasty or now more commonly vulvoplasty. This surgery consists of clitoroplasty, labiaplasty, and urethroplasty similar to other techniques; however, a neovaginal canal is not created, which precludes need for dilation and ability to have penetrative intercourse. This option is good for patients who have a history of pelvic radiation or surgery, those who do not want to or cannot dilate, those with multiple comorbidities, or those who do not desire a vaginal canal.[17] Health care providers should also understand that genital examinations can be triggering for transgender patients. The physical examination of the perineum and genitalia should be performed with sensitivity and patients should redress before any important surgical discussion takes place.[18] During the examination it is important to note the laxity and amount of the penile shaft and scrotal skin, density of pubic hair, presence of circumcision, ability to retract the foreskin if uncircumcised, scarring or inflammation of the glans, presence of inguinal hernias, and scars or lesions that jeopardize the skin graft. Consistent, long-term dilatation is crucial to the success of full-depth vaginoplasty and patients should be well aware of this commitment before surgery. Pelvic floor health plays a key role in dilation success. In a 2018 study, 42% of transfemale patients who had preoperative pelvic floor examinations were found to have some level of pelvic floor dysfunction, suggesting that preoperative pelvic floor physical therapy may be useful in the long-term success of vaginoplasty.[19] In addition, as many as 64% of the transgender population report a history of sexual abuse.[20] It is well established in the cisgender population that a history of physical, sexual, and/or emotional abuse is associated with pelvic floor dysfunction.[21] Patients should have the opportunity during their preoperative courses to discuss any prior sexual trauma and attend preoperative pelvic floor physical therapy. This issue is another example of how a multidisciplinary team is the best model to optimize patient outcomes. Patients should be educated on the need for postoperative speculum examinations and how to assert agency during such examinations. Other factors that may contribute to pelvic floor dysfunction are restroom insecurity (and therefore avoiding public restrooms), the act of tucking the scrotum and penis, and the use of antiandrogens. Exogenous estrogen is stopped 2 weeks before surgery to decrease the risk of perioperative thrombosis. Bowel preparation is initiated 2 days before surgery to maximize healing in the setting of an intraoperative rectal injury and immediate repair during the neovaginal canal dissection.

Surgical Principles: Vaginoplasty

Penile-inversion vaginoplasty begins with harvesting of the scrotal graft and then isolation of the testicles for orchiectomy. The scrotal graft (Fig. 1) will be anastomosed to the penile skin to create a closed tube that will line the neovaginal canal. Dissection of the neovaginal canal begins by palpating the central tendon and dissecting toward the central tendon by proceeding along the inferior border of the urethral bulb. A urinary catheter or Lowsley retractor is placed in the bladder to help guide dissection and rotate the prostate anteriorly. Sharp dissection is continued to the prostate, at which point Denonvilliers fascia is identified. Once the proper space is identified, the neovaginal canal is created by bluntly opening up this potential space using Haney retractors anteriorly and posteriorly (Video 1). The length of the neovaginal canal is limited by the peritoneal reflection. Hemostasis is established and the neovaginal canal is temporarily packed with gauze. Penile disassembly begins with degloving the penis proximal to the corona to create an open-end, superiorly based tubular skin flap. Component separation of the penis involves separation of the urethra from the corpus cavernosum, removal of the corpus cavernosum, and preservation of the glans penis with the neurovascular bundle. The glans is reduced and shaped into a neoclitoris. The

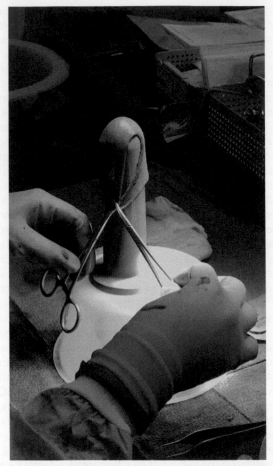

Fig. 1. Preparing the scrotal graft for anastomosis to the penile skin flap.

neurovascular bundle is then folded onto itself and placed at the level of the adductor longus tendons to properly position the clitoris on the vulva. The penile flap and scrotal skin graft construct is inverted and advanced into the neovaginal canal. New vaginal packing with antibiotic ointment is packed tightly into the canal to help bolster the graft to the neovaginal wall. A clitoral hood is then created from the prepuce skin. The remaining lateral scrotal tissue is transformed into labia majora (**Figs. 2–4**). The urethra is then transected to the level of the perineum and inset between the clitoris at the anterior vaginal wall, to allow sitting micturition. At the end of the procedure, the labia majora are sewn together to secure the vaginal packing in the neovaginal canal because it stays in place along with the urethral catheter and drains for 6 days postoperatively.

Patients who undergo full-depth vaginoplasty must commit to vaginal dilation to prevent neovaginal stenosis. Neovaginal stenosis is the narrowing or shortening of the vaginal canal over time, which greatly interferes with dilation and sexual activity. Dilation starts once the neovaginal packing is removed and must be continued according to the recommended schedule, with several (4) daily dilations during recovery to a maintenance schedule of once daily after about a year. Dilation is the insertion of a

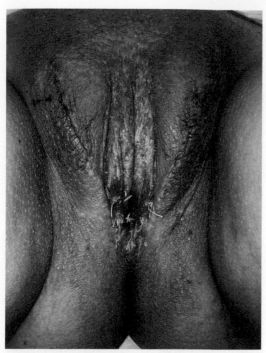

Fig. 2. Vaginoplasty; postoperative week 2.

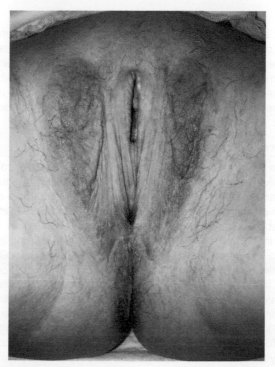

Fig. 3. Vaginoplasty: postoperative month 3.

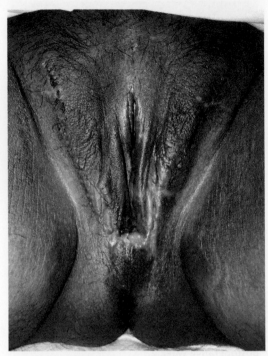

Fig. 4. Vaginoplasty: 6 weeks postoperative.

lubricated dilator into the neovaginal canal with sustained pressure on the vaginal apex for a period of at least 15 to 20 minutes. Failure to do so can result in neovaginal canal stenosis. Neovaginal stenosis requires additional surgery to recreate the neovaginal canal. In some cases, the secondary vaginoplasty is achieved by the addition of skin grafts to the stenosed portion of the canal, but may also require a complex reconstruction with either an intestinal or peritoneal flap to reestablish the entire length of the neovaginal canal.

Vaginoplasty Potential Complications

Granulation tissue is common postoperatively and is easily managed in the outpatient setting (**Fig. 5**). Silver nitrate treatments to the affected areas at regular intervals promote healing. Granulation tissue may present as painful dilatations or malodorous or bloody discharge on the dilator or pads. Patients should be educated on signs and symptoms so that they can be proactive about seeking evaluation. It is important to identify and treat intravaginal granulation tissue to prevent scarring and loss of depth. Fistulas are also a known complication of feminizing vaginoplasty. During neovaginal canal dissection, injury to the adjacent urethra, bladder anteriorly, or rectum posteriorly can occur. If the injury is identified at the time of surgery, it is repaired in layers. However, a urethrovaginal or rectovaginal fistula can form if an intraoperative injury is not identified or the repair fails. The overall incidence of rectoneovaginal fistula in a recent large cohort study of 1082 postoperative transwomen was 1.2%.[22] Although the risk is low, fistulas can have catastrophic effects on surgical outcomes and require additional surgery to repair. Rectoneovaginal fistulas typically present as foul-smelling discharge, stool, or gas coming from the neovaginal canal. Diagnosis can be made in

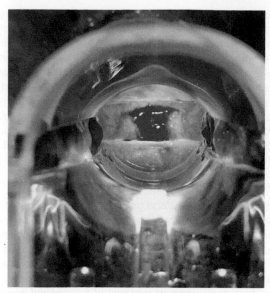

Fig. 5. Granulation tissue at the apex of the neovaginal canal.

the clinic by speculum and rectal examination to identify the site of the fistula. A diverting colostomy alone may lead to fistula closure; however, most patients with a recto-neovaginal fistula require definitive repair after the diverting colostomy. Urethroneovaginal fistulas present as urine coming from the neovaginal canal. Small urethroneovaginal fistulas may heal spontaneously with urinary diversion. A suprapubic catheter can be inserted to divert urine from the lower urinary tract and therefore promote healing. Patients who require surgical repair typically have a suprapubic catheter for several weeks postoperatively to allow the repair to heal adequately.

Other urinary complications include urethral stricture and malposition of the urethra. Urethral strictures present as a narrowing or weakening of the urinary stream. Patients often report having to push to initiate urinary flow and the sensation of incomplete voiding. Strictures are most likely to occur at the urethral meatus. Urethral dilation has been shown to be ineffective and possibly damage vital tissue needed for repair, and therefore a primary surgical repair is recommended.

Patients should be able to easily sit to urinate without any urine spraying onto their clothes, legs, or over the toilet seat. A malpositioned urethra may result in difficulty voiding and further exacerbate bathroom insecurity. Surgical mobilization and repositioning of the urethra can redirect the urinary stream downward. Patients should be educated on proper bathroom hygiene to avoid urinary tract infections; for example, wiping front to back.

TRANSMASCULINE GENITOURINARY SURGERY
Preoperative Considerations

Transmasculine patients have 2 main options to consider for genitourinary surgery: metoidioplasty and phalloplasty. The decision as to which procedure is better suited to the patient is based on his goals of surgery, anatomy, and acceptance of risks and possible complications. The preoperative assessment should include a thorough discussion of the patient's surgical goals. The most common surgical goals include a desire to stand to urinate, achieve penetrative intercourse, and natural-appearing aesthetics. Because binary transition is not a requirement for surgery, individual goals of surgical transition should be carefully considered by the multidisciplinary team with the patient, and in accordance with WPATH SOC. For example, some patients experience dysphoria surrounding urination and desire urethral lengthening to allow standing micturition, whereas others wish to avoid any potential urinary complications. Other patients may forgo vaginectomy for various reasons. Patient goals should be carefully considered with surgical feasibility and risks in mind. For instance, urethral lengthening without vaginectomy increases the risk of urethrocutaneous fistula,[23] and is generally not recommended. The approach and staging to transmasculine surgeries can vary but are generally referred to as a simple metoidioplasty, complex metoidioplasty, and single-stage or 2-stage phalloplasty.

Surgical Principles: Metoidioplasty

A simple metoidioplasty is a single-stage gender-affirming surgery for transmasculine patients that releases the hormonally enlarged clitoris by dividing the suspensory ligament that anchors the clitoris to the pubic bone. This procedure allows the shaft of the neophallus to be released from its superior attachment to give a slightly lengthened appearance. A complex or full metoidioplasty includes the procedure described earlier with the addition of a vaginectomy and urethral lengthening.

Vaginectomy involves destruction or removal of the vaginal mucosa through excision or electrocautery followed by colpocleisis. Urethral lengthening is the creation of a neourethra between the native meatus to the tip of the neophallus (enlarged clitoris). Local flaps, such as labia minora tissue or vaginal mucosa, or grafts such as buccal grafts, can be used to create the neourethra. A suprapubic catheter is placed to divert the urinary stream for 3 to 4 weeks postoperatively, until the patient is able to void via urethra without complications. The ability to stand and urinate is generally attributed to the degree of clitoromegaly in response to testosterone supplementation and the ability of the patient's genital anatomy. Patients with higher BMI and fuller mons are less likely to have the protrusion of their neophallus to a degree that could be adequate for standing to urinate. Typically with a metoidioplasty, penetrative sex is not feasible unless there is a significant clitoromegaly caused by testosterone (**Fig. 6**).

Metoidioplasty Potential Complications

Complications of metoidioplasty range from minor issues to those requiring urethral reconstruction. Minor complications include wound dehiscence and urinary tract infection. Voiding trial via neourethra can be attempted when swelling has improved. After 1 week of reliable urination without difficulty or urethral complications, the suprapubic catheter may be removed. Roughly 30% of metoidioplasty patients develop urethral complications.[24] A urethrocutaneous fistula typically manifests as a split stream or leakage of urine along the penile shaft but may also present in the perineum or anterior intergluteal cleft (**Fig. 7**). In this case, the voiding trial is delayed and the bladder is continuously drained by the suprapubic catheter. Most fistulas heal without intervention over time and urinary diversion. Large or persistent fistulas are best repaired, typically with the addition of a hairless skin graft or buccal mucosa.[25] After the suprapubic catheter is removed and patients are urinating through their neourethras, they should be made aware of symptoms of urinary obstruction, most commonly caused by urethral stricture. A urethral stricture is a narrowing of the urethra, and is most commonly located at the anastomosis between the native urethra and the neourethra. Urinary retention is a medical emergency and requires emergent drainage through urethral catheter placement or suprapubic catheter replacement.

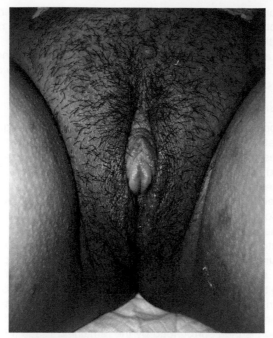

Fig. 6. Postoperative metoidioplasty without scrotoplasty.

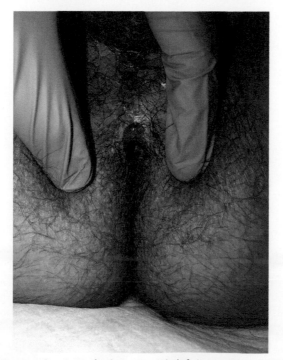

Fig. 7. Urethrocutaneous fistula in the intergluteal cleft in a postoperative metoidioplasty.

Stricture repair can typically be managed with an outpatient or overnight procedure. Patients may elect to have a scrotoplasty at the same time as the metoidioplasty or after several months when the swelling has resolved.

Scrotoplasty is achieved by elevating labia majora then folding and medializing the tissue to create a scrotum. Testicular implants are usually placed in a delayed setting to lessen the risk of implant exposure and wound dehiscence.

Surgical Principles: Phalloplasty

The goal of phalloplasty is to construct an aesthetic penis with erogenous and tactile sensation and that allows standing urination and penetrative intercourse. There are various techniques and staging for phalloplasty, and thus a 1-size-fits-all approach is not encouraged. The radial forearm and the ALT are the 2 preferred donor sites because the tissue can be reinnervated. Other donor sites include the latissimus dorsi myocutaneous free flap, lower abdominal pedicled flap, and osteocutaneous fibula free flap. These donor sites lack sensory innervation sufficient to facilitate erogenous sensation in the neophallus and are generally not recommended. The patient's goals as well as his anatomy help guide the choice of donor site. Most commonly, the neophallus and neourethra are created from an RFFF. The RFFF approach is widely preferred among surgeons because it allows the construction of a sensate penis and neourethra in the same setting. The thinness of the skin and subcutaneous tissue allows the creation of the neourethral tube within the neophallus at the time of the initial operation, also commonly referred to as a double-tube, where the first tube is the skin-lined urethra, which is then surrounded by the remaining tissue (**Figs. 8** and **9**). The main drawback is the visible, nearly circumferential forearm scar. Patients who wish to avoid forearm scarring, have a history of prohibitive forearm trauma, or have radial

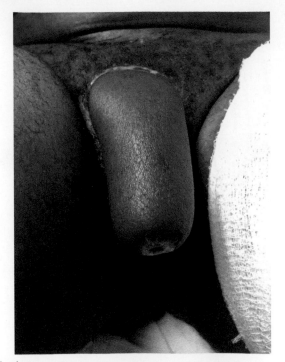

Fig. 8. RFFF phalloplasty.

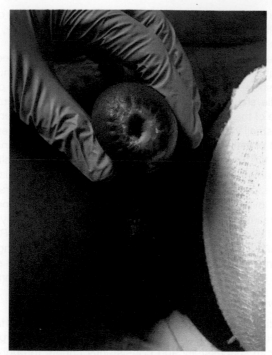

Fig. 9. RFFF phalloplasty: urethral meatus.

artery dominance may choose pedicled ALT (**Fig. 10**). The thigh often provides more bulk to the phallus and sometimes more length, and has the advantage of being a more easily concealed donor site.

However, because of the increased thickness of the thigh tissue, ALT can rarely be double tubed. If the patient wishes to be able to stand to urinate, secondary urethroplasty has to be performed to construct the urethra. Phalloplasty from ALT typically requires more surgeries than RFFF phalloplasty to complete phalloplasty. These procedures may include glansplasty and debulking via liposuction to achieve a diameter

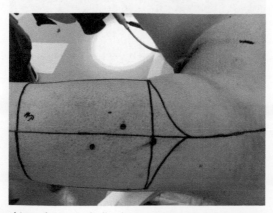

Fig. 10. Surgical markings for ALT phalloplasty.

reasonable for penetrative intercourse. In addition, ALT phalloplasty carries higher risk for urethral complications. To cover the forearm or thigh donor site, a split-thickness skin graft is taken from the uninvolved thigh (**Fig. 11**).

Electrolysis is required on the surface of the donor site that will become the urethra to avoid complications such as urinary obstruction from hair accumulation and stone formation. It is also recommended that patients have electrolysis on areas that will become the penile shaft, because cisgender male penises generally do not grow hair past the base of the shaft. The aim of the surgery is to create an aesthetic, functional penis, and small variances such as hair growth can trigger gender dysphoria.

For sensation, 1 of the 2 dorsal clitoral nerves is coapted to the nerve from the donor flap (**Figs. 12** and **13**). The clitoris is buried at the base of the neophallus or exposed at its ventral base. When the sensation is restored to the neophallus, which typically takes about a year, penile implants can be inserted to allow penetrative intercourse.

Phalloplasty recovery is a challenging process that requires coordination of the multidisciplinary team with the patient and the patient's support system. The donor site and skin graft site require wound care. Patients who elect an RFFF phalloplasty need several weeks of hand occupational therapy to reduce swelling and help regain full function. Complications in phalloplasty are common. A 2018 study found that roughly 31.5% of RFFF phalloplasty patients experience urinary complications.[26]

Phalloplasty Potential Complications

Similar to metoidioplasty, urethral strictures are common, occurring in up to 57% of patients.[27] A suprapubic catheter is inserted at the time of surgery and remains until the patient can successfully and consistently urinate through the neophallus. The urethra after phalloplasty is composed of 3 main sections: the native urethra, the fixed urethra (pars fixa made during the urethral lengthening portion), and the pendulous urethra (pars pendulous, urethra made from the flap tissue). Typically strictures arise at the anastomosis between these sections. Narrowing can also

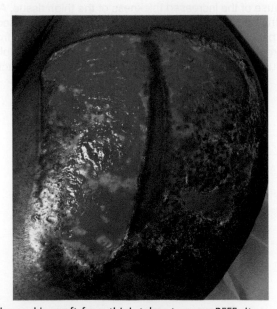

Fig. 11. Split-thickness skin graft from thigh taken to cover RFFF site.

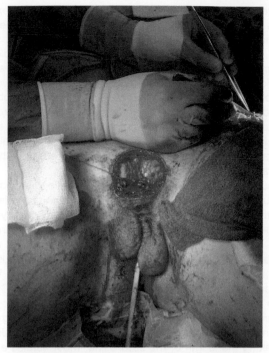

Fig. 12. ALT phalloplasty: surgeons working on harvesting ALT donor site. Clitoris is isolated and coapted. Patient had a previous scrotoplasty and did not elect urethroplasty; therefore, the catheter is in the native urethra. This patient sits to urinate and simply lifts the scrotum.

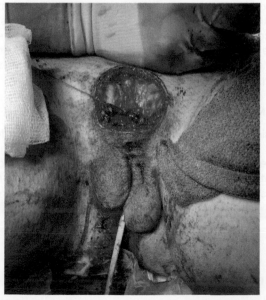

Fig. 13. Closer view of ALT phalloplasty procedure. Note the suture placed in the clitoris, which will be buried within the phallus to facilitate erogenous sensation postoperatively.

occur at the urethra meatus at the tip of the neophallus. Approximately 40% to 60% of strictures occur at the level of the pars fixa and pars pendulans urethral anastomosis. Strictures typically occur at 2 to 6 months after surgery but can occur even later than 1 year.[27] Patients report obstructive voiding symptoms, such as weak urinary stream, incomplete emptying, and increased frequency and urgency. Strictures need to be addressed expediently to avoid an emergent situation of complete obstruction. When patients present with obstructive symptoms, they should undergo cystoscopy and/or retrograde urethrogram to assess for urethral disorder. Patients with impending urinary retention should receive a suprapubic tube for urinary diversion. Urethral dilation is generally a temporizing measure. Most patients need to undergo a definitive urethroplasty with or without skin or buccal graft.[27]

Urethrocutaneous (UC) fistula is the most common phalloplasty complication and is most likely to occur just proximal to a stricture[27] because this area is poorly vascularized. In the urethral lengthening portion of phalloplasty, many layers of well-vascularized tissue from the vestibule can be used to promote urethral integrity, if vaginectomy and colpocleisis is performed. Phalloplasty without vaginectomy has been shown to have a significantly higher rate of urethrocutaneous fistula because this tissue is not available to reinforce the urethra. Therefore, it is recommended that patients undergoing phalloplasty also elect vaginectomy.[28] UC fistulas are fairly straightforward to diagnose and typically occur soon after surgery. Patients report a split stream of urine while voiding, incomplete voiding, and leaking of fluid. Physical examination can reveal a visible fistula at the base of the neophallus, but they can occur anywhere along the length of the suture line. Most fistulas are small and can heal spontaneously. Large fistulas need surgical repair with or without augmentation with skin or buccal grafts.

SUMMARY

Gender-affirming genitourinary surgery represents a pivotal moment in gender transition and can greatly improve quality of life. Risks and complications should be extensively discussed so that patient expectations are reasonable and the patients are fully informed. The use of a multidisciplinary team of surgeons, endocrinologists, primary care providers, mental health therapists, social workers, and physical therapists is key to optimizing patient outcomes and overall care.

CLINICS CARE POINTS

- Penile inversion vaginoplasty is the most common approach for male to female transition.
- Fertility preservation should be discussed at the time of surgical consult.
- Complex metoidioplasty typically does not facilitate standing micturition.
- Electrology is the superior method of hair removal prior to surgery.

DISCLOSURE

No disclosures.

SUPPLEMENTARY DATA

Supplementary data related to this article can be found online at https://doi.org/10.1016/j.cpha.2020.11.010.

REFERENCES

1. Stroumsa D. The state of transgender health care: policy, law, and medical frameworks. Am J Public Health 2014;104(3):e31–8.
2. Dowshen NL, Christensen J, Gruschow SM. Health insurance coverage of recommended gender-affirming health care services for transgender youth: shopping online for coverage information. Transgend Health 2019;4(1):131–5.
3. James SE, Herman JL, Rankin S, et al. The report of the 2015 U.S. Transgender survey. Washington, DC: National Center for Transgender Equality; 2016.
4. Pariser JJ, Kim N. Transgender vaginoplasty: techniques and outcomes. Transl Androl Urol 2019;8(3):241–7.
5. Ting J, Bowers M. Penile inversion vaginoplasty. In: Schechter L, editor. Gender confirmation surgery. Cham (Switzerland): Springer; 2020.
6. Melich JG, Marecik S. Intestinal vaginoplasty. In: Schechter L, editor. Gender confirmation surgery. Cham (Switzerland): Springer; 2020.
7. Mhatre P, Mhatre J, Sahu R. New laparoscopic peritoneal pull-through vaginoplasty technique. J Hum Reprod Sci 2014;7(3):181–6.
8. Perovic SV, Djordjevic ML. Metoidioplasty: a variant of phalloplasty in female transsexuals. BJU Int 2003;92(9):981–5.
9. Schechter LS, Safa B. Introduction to phalloplasty. Clin Plast Surg 2018;45(3): 387–9.
10. World Professional Association for Transgender Health. Standards of care for the health of transsexual, transgender, and gender-nonconforming people. 7th version 2009. p. 54-65.
11. Berli JU, Knudson G, Fraser L, et al. What surgeons need to know about gender confirmation surgery when providing care for transgender individuals: a review. JAMA Surg 2017;152(4):394–400.
12. Lindström D, Sadr Azodi O, Wladis A, et al. Effects of a perioperative smoking cessation intervention on postoperative complications: a randomized trial. Ann Surg 2008;248(5):739–45.
13. Hembree Wylie C, Cohen-Kettenis PT, Gooren L, et al. Endocrine treatment of gender-dysphoric/gender-incongruent persons: an endocrine society clinical practice guideline. J Clin Endocrinol Metab 2017;102(11):3869–903.
14. Light AD, Obedin-Maliver J, Sevelius JM, et al. Transgender men who experienced pregnancy after female-to-male gender transitioning. Obstet Gynecol 2014;124:1120–7.
15. ASRM. Fertility preservation in patients undergoing gonadotoxic therapy or gonadectomy: a committee opinion. Fertil Steril 2019;112(6):1022–33.
16. Ainsworth A, Allyse M, Khan Z. Fertility preservation for transgender individuals: a review. Mayo Clin Proc 2020;95(4):784–92.
17. Jiang D, Witten J, Berli J, et al. Does depth matter? factors affecting choice of vulvoplasty over vaginoplasty as gender-affirming genital surgery for transgender women. J Sex Med 2018;15(6):902–6.
18. Cavanaugh T, Hopwood R, Lambert C. Informed consent in the medical care of transgender and gender-nonconforming patients. AMA J Ethics 2016;18(11): 1147–55.
19. Jiang DD, Gallagher S, Burchill L, et al. Implementation of a pelvic floor physical therapy program for transgender women undergoing gender-affirming vaginoplasty. Obstet Gynecol 2019;133(5):1003–11.

20. Grant Jaime M, Mottet Lisa A, Tanis Justin, et al. Injustice at every turn: a report of the national transgender discrimination survey. Washington, DC: National Center for Transgender Equality and National Gay and Lesbian Task Force; 2011.
21. Cichowski SB, Dunivan GC, Komesu YM, et al. Sexual abuse history and pelvic floor disorders in women. South Med J 2013;106(12):675–8.
22. Horbach SE, Bouman MB, Smit JM, et al. Outcome of vaginoplasty in male-to-female transgenders: a systematic review of surgical techniques. J Sex Med 2015;12(6):1499–512.
23. Chesson RR, Gilbert DA, Jordan GH, et al. The role of colpocleisis with urethral lengthening in transsexual phalloplasty. Am J Obstet Gynecol 1996;175(6):1443–50.
24. Djordjevic ML, Stojanovic B, Bizic M. Metoidioplasty: techniques and outcomes. Transl Androl Urol 2019;8(3):248–53.
25. Chen ML, Reyblat P, Poh MM, et al. Overview of surgical techniques in gender-affirming genital surgery. Transl Androl Urol 2019;8(3):191–208.
26. Ascha M, Massie JP, Morrison SD, et al. Outcomes of single stage phalloplasty by pedicled anterolateral thigh flap versus radial forearm free flap in gender confirming surgery. J Urol 2018;199(1):206–14.
27. Jun MS, Santucci RA. Urethral stricture after phalloplasty. Transl Androl Urol 2019;8(3):266–72.
28. Al-Tamimi M, Pigot GL, van der Sluis WB, et al. Colpectomy significantly reduces the risk of urethral fistula formation after urethral lengthening in transgender men. J Urol 2018;200(6):1315–22.

Printed and bound by CPI Group (UK) Ltd, Croydon, CR0 4YY

03/10/2024

01040399-0016